José David Rodríguez Martínez

A Wearable Platform for Patient Monitoring during Mass Casualty Incidents

A Wearable Platform for Patient Monitoring during Mass Casualty Incidents

by

José David Rodríguez Martínez

KIT Scientific Publishing

Karlsruher Institut für Technologie
Institut für Technik der Informationsverarbeitung

A Wearable Platform for Patient Monitoring during Mass Casualty Incidents

Zur Erlangung des akademischen Grades eines Doktor-Ingenieurs von der Fakultät für Elektrotechnik und Informationstechnik des Karlsruher Instituts für Technologie (KIT) genehmigte Dissertation

von M. Sc. José David Rodríguez Martínez aus Mexiko-Stadt, Mexiko

Tag der mündlichen Prüfung: 16. Dezember 2014
Gutachter: Prof. Dr. rer. nat. Wilhelm Stork, Prof. Dr. Stefan Nickel

Impressum

KIT Scientific Publishing

Karlsruher Institut für Technologie (KIT)
KIT Scientific Publishing
Straße am Forum 2
D-76131 Karlsruhe

KIT Scientific Publishing is a registered trademark of Karlsruhe Institute of Technology.
Reprint using the book cover is not allowed.

www.ksp.kit.edu

Print on Demand 2018 – Gedruckt auf FSC-zertifiziertem Papier

ISBN 978-3-7315-0486-3
DOI 10.5445/KSP/1000051989

to Sofía and Santiago David

Acknowledgements

This dissertation is the result of my years as a research scientist in the Department of Embedded Systems and Sensors Engineering at the *FZI Forschungszentrum Informatik am Karlsruher Institut für Technologie*. The realization of this work would not have been possible without the invaluable support and help of many people.

In the first place, I want to thank Prof. Dr. rer. nat. Wilhelm Stork for the given opportunity and guidance. He has been a continuous source of inspiration, motivation and strength for the conclusion of this dissertation. I want to specially thank Prof. Dr.-Ing. Stefan Nickel for having taken part as coreferent and for supporting the submission of this work.

As well, I thank all my colleagues for the teamwork and for the infinite and creative discussions. Above all, I thank my advisors Dr.-Ing. Stephan Heuer and Prof. Dr.-Ing. Christophe Kunze for the given trust, the constant impulse and the inspiring work atmosphere. For the friendly enviroment, I thank my colleagues Dr.-Ing. Bruno Rosales, Fernando Sánchez, Javier Parada and Imanol Bernabeu. Additionally, I thank all the involved students that, under my advice and with their work and commitment, provide new and relevant developments for this dissertation.

I want to sincerly thank my sister Denise and my parents Laura and David for their constant love, and for showing that despite the distance they are always there for me.

Finally, I do not have words to express my infinite thanks to my wife Carolina, her support and endless patience made possible this work.

Stuttgart, May 4th, 2015
José David Rodríguez Martínez

Zusammenfassung

Die Sichtung von Opfern bei einem Massenanfall von Verletzten stellt die Rettungskräfte im Einsatz vor eine sehr große Herausforderung. Dieser Aufwand kann mit der Einführung von eingebetteten mit Netzwerktechnologien und automatischen Systemen zur Entscheidungsunterstützung enorm verringert werden.

Intelligente Algorithmen können mithilfe von physiologischen Daten dabei helfen, die am schwersten verletzten Opfer einzuordnen und zu erkennen. Sichtungsinformationen, bzw. die Priorisierung von Opfern, sind für die Planung von medizinischer Versorgung und Krankenhaustransporten massgebend.

Die Analyse von gängigen Sichtungsprozessen und Gespräche mit Fachpersonal haben ergeben, dass die momentan verwendeten Methoden und Geräte rudimentär sind; ein Mangel an Informationen und die regelmässige Aktualisierung von Informationen stellt nach wie vor eine Hürde für das Personal von Rettungsleitstellen dar. Momentan werden bei Rettungseinsätzen Papierkarten und analoge Kommunikationsgeräte verwendet, die bei der Sichtung und Organisation am Einsatzort nicht sehr effektiv sind.

Forschungsprojekte in den letzten zehn Jahren haben ergeben, dass die Einführung von neuen Informations- und Kommunikationstechnologien den Dokumentations- und Kommunikationsprozess vor Ort beschleunigen könnte. Laut Experten für Rettungseinsätze gibt es in diesem Bereich jedoch noch Verbesserungsmöglichkeiten. In dieser Dissertation wird eine neue, sensorbasierte Sichtungsplattform dargestellt, deren wichtigste Funktion die Verbindung von verschiedenen Sensoren und Kommunikationstechnologien in einem tragbaren Gerät ist. Dieses neue Gerät soll die Rettungseinheiten bei der taktischen Planung des Einsatzes unterstützen.

Für eine stichhaltige Definition der neuen Sensorplattform wurden zunächst häufig verwendete Sichtungsprozesse analysiert. Die ersten Indikatoren bei einer Sichtung sind Bewusstsein und körperliche Einschränkung, gefolgt vom Atmungs- und Kreislaufzustand. Der neue, automatische Sichtungsansatz basiert auf der automatischen Erkennung und Analyse dieser physiologischen Parameter.

Eine am Handgelenk zu befestigende Plattform wird mit den benötigten Überwachungsmodulen ausgestattet und um drahtlose Kommunikations- und Lokalisierungsfunktionen erweitert. Diese Plattform erstellt eine automatische Analyse und übermittelt der Rettungsleitstelle den Status und die Lokalisierung am Einsatzort. Die Regeln zur Evaluierung von physiologischen Parametern wurden mithilfe von Experten entwickelt. Das Ziel hierbei war die automatische Unterscheidung, ob der Zustand des Opfers kritisch ist oder nicht.

Diese Dissertation behandelt die Implementierung und Evaluierung der neuen tragbaren Überwachungsplattform und überprüft die Hypothese, dass mit diesem System entscheidende Patientendaten erfasst werden können, um den taktischen Einsatz von Sanitätern vor Ort bei einem MANV zu verbessern. Die experimentellen Daten zur Validierung der Plattform wurden bei Notfallübungen und bei neunzig echten Notfalleinsätzen erhoben.

Abstract

The triage of victims during mass casualty incidents represents an enormous effort for the rescue personnel involved. This effort can be effectively reduced with the introduction of networked embedded technologies and automated decision support systems.

Based on physiological data, intelligent algorithms can assist with the classification and recognition of the most severely impaired victims. The triage information or the prioritization of victims is crucial for the management of the medical assistance and the hospital transportation.

An analysis of current triage procedures and discussions with practitioners reveals that actual methods and tools are rudimentary; the lack of accurate information and continuous information update is still an obstacle for rescue managers. Paper cards and analog communication devices are the actual rescue means, and they do not assist the triage and the organization in the field.

During the last decade, research projects have shown how the introduction of new information and communications technologies represent an opportunity to accelerate the documentation and communication process on-site. However, experts from emergency fields indicate that there is still room for improvement. This dissertation presents a new sensor-based triage platform where the main proposal is to join different sensor and communications technologies into a portable device. This new device must be able to assist the rescue units along with the tactical planning of the operation.

For a valid definition of a new sensor platform, commonly applied triage procedures were firstly analyzed. Consciousness and disability are identified as the first triage indicators, followed by the respiration and the circulation condition. The new automatic triage approach is based on the automatic sensing and analysis of these physiological parameters.

A wrist wearable platform is integrated with the necessary monitoring modules; additionally it is extended with wireless communication and localization functions.This platform automatically features the analysis and communicates the status and localization to the rescue managers at the incident area. The rules to evaluate the physiological parameters were defined together with practitioners, where the goal was the automated distinction between critical and non-critical victims.

This dissertation discusses the implementation and the evaluation of the new wearable monitoring platform. It presents and test the hypothesis that, with such a system, it is possible to collect sense-making patient data to support the tactical planning of first response during MCI. Experimental data for platform validation were recorded during emergency drills and also during ninety real emergency shifts.

Contents

1 Introduction

The German Institute for Standardization (DIN), in the norm DIN 13050, defines a mass casualty incident (MCI) as an emergency with a large number of injured or ill and other affected people. This type of emergency cannot be managed with the available and usable provisions of ambulant relief services within the operation area [BKH+09].

In the last decades, reports on natural and technological disasters have been a constant in the news media around the globe. The social attention constantly focuses on disaster events. A continuous changing demographical landscape, increasing extreme environmental conditions, the rise of urbanization, and permanent terrorism menace, increase the vulnerability of the society to disasters, see Figure 1.1. These events represent a breakpoint in the civilian security, and they are to be attended by the authorities.

A disaster event or a mass casualty incident (MCI) represents an undesired event for the social system. As defined by United Nations (UN), a disaster is a serious disruption of the function of a society. It causes widespread human, material, or environmental losses, which exceed the ability of the affected society to react using only its resources [U.N92].

Available reports from the World Health Organization (WHO) indicate a radical increment on the amount of disasters between the 1990 and 2000 decades. However, in the last decade, the number of disasters has remained constant. Each year, disaster events result into a mean of two hundred million of victims, see figure 1.2 [WDH+10].

1.1 Motivation

When an MCI occurs, the objective of first response and emergency relief organizations is to apply as fast as possible efficient relief mechanisms.

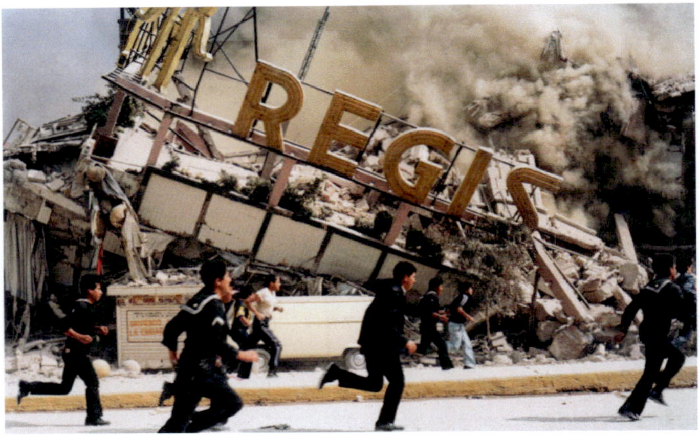

Figure 1.1: Mexico City earthquake, 8.1 on the Richter scale, September 1985 (http://www.spiegel.de/einestages/erdbeben-in-mexiko-a-949141.html)

They have to achieve the tactical planning to provide proper medical care to the affected people and to preserve as many lives as possible.

The magnitude of MCI sets an enormous challenge to the emergency organizations since they are normally outnumbered by the amount of casualties. In order to deliver emergency relief and stabilize the scenario, a well-organized supply service is a mandate. The organization of the first respond relies on the available communications technology and the information management.

The demand for accurate information on the field is extreme. A tactical management during the rescue operation is based on the rapid characterization of the scenario. The rescue plan requires to finding and to supporting as soon as possible the most impaired victims and tracking the progress or deterioration of all the affected individuals.

In the first place, paramedics and prehospital emergency doctors (PED) work together as data miners. They assess the victim's condition and determine the attention priority for each of them. They inform this data to the incident officer to support him with the management of medical resources, transport and communication with hospitals.

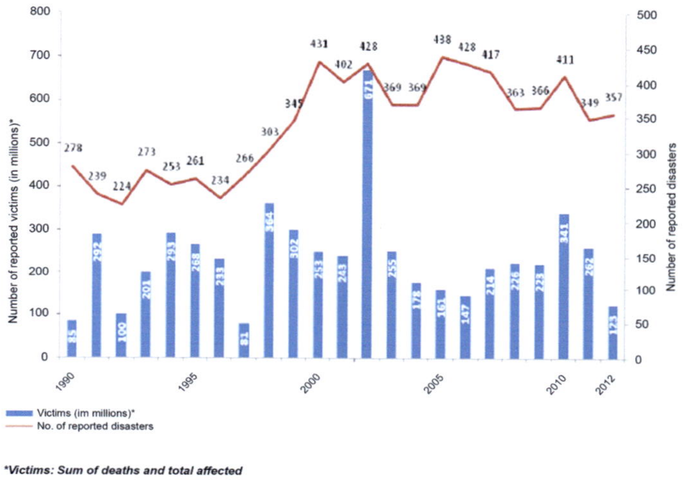

Figure 1.2: Reported disasters from last 2 decades

Lessons learned has shown that the performance of actual emergency information and communication systems has been a long-standing issue of concern. They are rudimentary and does not fulfill the demand of information on the field. Besides that, they increase the level of uncertainty, generating more chaos and stress. Moreover, civilian and commercial communication infrastructure does not represent a solution for the first responder's necessities. MCI set specific requirements for the implementation of ICT on the field [Vem04] [NG99b].

Latest advances in ICT, mainly from the area of embedded systems, autonomous sensor networks, mobile computing and expert systems in telemedicine represent a potential success opportunity to support the MCI management. Research from the last ten years shows how the introduction of newest ICT can improve the communication, information, and documentation processes radically. New ICT can support the incident officers to track the scenario in real-time. Information is automatically displayed on the screen, supporting the decision-making process.

This dissertation continues the research work around the application of ICT with the aim to support the incident officers with the planning of the first respond activities.

1.2 Objective and Own Contribution

The objective of this dissertation is to continue the introduction and optimization of new ICT platforms into the first response process and to assess the impact and challenges of these new platforms at MCI. The main goal is to support the tactical planning of the rescue operation and to provide the first responder with sense-making information at any time of the operation.

Accomplishment of such objectives demands the understanding and the analysis MCI management requirements. Thus, the collection and analysis of the requirements are based on a user-centered design approach. The conception and implementation of the new platform follow the guidelines of experts in the field.

This dissertation deals with the implementation of a wearable platform for the monitoring the classification of victims, being more important the automatic identification of the most impaired victims automatically.

This dissertation presents a new sensor-based portable platform. The platform extended with communication technologies, sensor and algorithms to assess the physiological condition of the patients automatically.

One of the main contributions is the validation of the new platform, testing the hypothesis, which states that is possible to support the MCI management with such a system. Tools and methods for the development and test of the new casualty monitoring platform are as well discussed.

This dissertation is the result of the work realized in two *Germany's Federal Ministry of Education and Reasearch (BMBF)* projects: ***MANET and SeCoServ2.***

1.3 Structure of the Dissertation

This dissertation follows the next structure:

In this first chapter, the introduction and motivation of the work are presented. A principles chapter introduces the required knowledge to understand the work presented in this dissertation, explaining the MCI management, the trauma physiology and the assessment of casualties. The third chapter discusses the state of the art and research. Chapter four explains the conception of the new. Chapter five describes the implementation of different prototypes. Chapter six depicts the evaluation of the new platform and validation of the casualty classification algorithm. Finally, chapter seven presents the conclusion and possible future work.

2 Principles

The management of a mass casualty incident (MCI) requires special medical logistics due to the extreme demand for information. It requires an efficient organizational structure, the application of standardized procedures, and the support of ad hoc information and communication systems.

Emergency commanders (EC) are the ones in charge to manage the provision of medical care. The scenario represents an organization and logistic challenge because the disproportion between the large number of patients and the available medical equipment and personnel [Cow82]. During MCI, medical resources need to be used to their extent to normalize the emergency scenario so that the largest amount of patients can receive personalized medical assistance. In consequence, an efficient distribution of health assistance requires primordially the medical categorization and prioritization of the patients. ECs needs, for the tactical planning, accurate information from the field, in order to answer: *who needs what, where is it needed and who needs it first* [MSYI11, oHS08]. The classification process to inform about the needs and status of the patients is commonly known as triage, and it is the primary responsibility of (PED)[KAGL96, Vem04].

This chapter introduces essential knowledge to simplify the understanding of the topic presented in this dissertation. It comprises fundamentals about the management of MCI and the commander structures. Proper advice towards the information and communication methods for data collection is also provided. Communication is primordial for the tactical planning of the operation and the provision of basic life support (BLS) and advanced life support (ALS). The term triage is in this chapter introduced, and it is a central topic of the scientific work covered in this dissertation. Triage is fundamental for the planning of the rescue operation. Its central role for the casualty management is depicted as well. Finally, a review of the trauma physiology and assessment is discussed, together with a review of the physiological systems normally affected during a trauma incident. Methods and tools to assess these systems, which is also relevant for the management of casualties, are also presented.

2.1 Management of Mass Casualty Incidents

During a relief operation, those with the management responsibilities should continually identify, refine, and validate resource requirements and the actual capacities. This process involves the accurate identification of what and how much, where and when it is necessary, and who will be receiving or using it. Identification of resources capacities includes medical equipment, supplies, facilities, and personnel or emergency response teams [CFY02, oHS08].

When an MCI occurs, the care provision depends on many variable conditions. The conditions influencing the relief process are the nature and causes of the urgency. The number of patients, the number of immediate rescue forces, availability of emergency transports affect directly the rescue logistics. Another determinant conditions are the weather conditions, distance to hospitals and accessibility for ambulances, helicopters, and first aid for the patients [CM05, PD10].

The tactical planning to approach the MCI scenario depends on the above conditions. Aside them, various technical factors are also taken into consideration, e.g. the need to set up a technical infrastructure to allow communication between the different actors. Communication is primordial to prepare the attention and transportation based on the medical assessment of the victims correctly. It also affects the coordination plan among various relief agencies, for example to define the correct disaster category, in order to trigger the fluent of rescue resources [RPA+09].

2.1.1 Organizational Rescue Structure and Logistics

During the course of the MCI, two organizational structures are mainly necessary: one dedicated to providing medical assistance to the victims and other to manage the technological aspects on the site. The establishment of the command center is required to enable an effective and efficient coordination between the different relief agencies and organizations. The success of the management relies on the communication and information systems, which requires a continuous flow of critical information. The interoperability between the management and response personnel and their affiliated organizations is only possible if they have a standard picture of the scenario [oHS08].

Awareness data is collected and informed to the control center, where it is continuously processed to manage and coordinate the whole process. The responsibilities of the command center rely only on the incident commander (IC) of the operation, see figure 2.1.

The IC coordinates the strategic communication between authorities, while relief agency leaders present at the incident scenario. The incident commander will support the communication between hospital concerning resource ordering, dispatching, and tracking; as well as the control the traffic and public around the affected area. Also, it is in charge of generating emergency alerts and warnings and of coordinating the press communication [CKGL04].

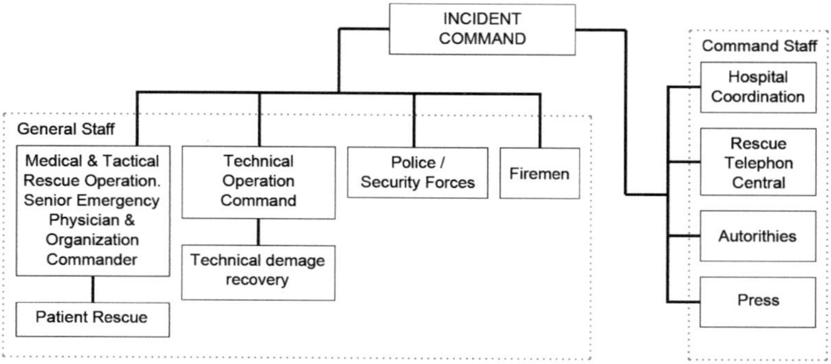

Figure 2.1: Incident command organization

Coordination of Medical Assistance

The public-safety answering point, a public emergency call center, is responsible to set the alarm and to trigger the rescue protocols concerning an MCI. It is in charge of informing to the relevant rescue services and the corresponding emergency experts, including PEDs and commanders. It also prevents the hospitals and the ambulance services about the incident. During the rescue operation, it will support the communication with the event area [GAR+05].

The medical assistance activities are managed by a medical incident officer (MIO). The MIO leads the activities of all the emergency medical forces on the site and takes control over the logistics and the medical supervision of the victims. In order to coordinate the medical operation, the MIO needs to estimate the urgency of the situation[GAR+05].

At the tactical level, it is necessary to establish first the kind of disaster, the type of injuries and illness. Also, important is to determine the number of injured and ill, the impact of the damage and identify potential hazards that could increment the disaster. On the other hand, the MIO needs to determine its personnel and material capacity, as well the nearby stationary treatment capacity.

Towards the planning and allocation of resources, the MIO requires the precise classification of the patients depending on the severity of their conditions. This information helps the MIO to plan efficiently and prioritize the provision of medical assistance.

The MIO establishes the treatment procedures and sets a priority for the victim's transportation to the hospitals. Based on the situational and patient information he plans and delegates different medical tasks to the paramedics. He determines the number and type of transport units, defines the demand for resources, such as medical equipment and medicaments, and documents the rescue operation continually. The MIO also needs to act as consultant or mediator, in case of doubts or controversial issues, regarding regular relief assistance arises [GAR+07].

Another important management function is the planning of the medical assistance activities. The ambulance incident officer (AIO) is in charge to coordinate them. The primary task is to achieve the targets defined by the MIO. This officer is in charge of gathering and presenting to the MIO the tactical information, to set up the treatment and transportation zone, and to coordinate the information flow between paramedics and the MIO [Vem04].

The mission of the MIO and the AIO is to provide adequate medical assistance and to avoid the collapse of nearby clinics. Instead, they secure the individualized support of the patients, dispatching the victims to specialized hospitals placed in a bigger radius.

Execution of Medical Assistance

The rescue team, composed mainly by PEDs and paramedics, executes the required medical actions. Four stages define the distribution of medical assistance [PRS07], see Figure 2.2. This division defines specific tasks for each phase and facilitates the organization of the rescue team. Following the description of Peters et al. in [PRS07], the four phases are:

- Phase 1: Arrival to the incident area und fast assessment of victims
- Phase 2: Categorization and prioritization of the victims
- Phase 3: Medical handling of each victim
- Phase 4: Transport of victims to the hospitals

Phase 1 - Arrival to the incident area

At the arrival to the incident area, a site recognition is first performed to clean the area, avoid possible hazards and reduce the danger. Then the rescue team starts assessing simple physiological functions of the victims. If necessary, first aid actions are applied to recover and assured vital functions. This process is the same for each victim and lasts in most of the cases typically less than two minutes per victim.

A fast assessment of vital functions allows a pre-categorization of the victims. A general overview of the patient's condition represents the first tactical information to the MIO and helps him to have a general view of the incident scenario. With this information, it can start estimating the acquisition and allocation of resources. Provision of BLS starts in this phase. ALS can only start when the diagnose, and type of treatment are specified.

Phase 2 - Categorization and prioritization of victims

The provision of individualized and medical assistance requires, after stabilizing the vital signs of the emergency patients; a detailed diagnose. A practical assistance is only possible if, apart from the number of victims, the nature and severity of its condition is determined. For the provision of care, it is necessary to specify the type of emergency, e.g.: pediatric, gynecologist, internal or surgical, traumatological, thermal, toxicological, etc. Aside the emergency type definition, the patient is categorized and prioritized depending on the severity of its injuries and illness. Only a PED is allowed to perform the categorization of the victims.

Phase 3 - Medical handling of victims

Based on the diagnosis and priority information of the patient, the paramedics set an on-site treatment area. There, the patients are sorted depending on the category of their condition. The MIO plans the treatment area, where he supports the allocation of the treatment and medicaments, as well as the preparation of the victims for transportation.Based on the diagnosis and priority information of the patient, the paramedics set an on-site treatment area. ALS actions starts in this phase.

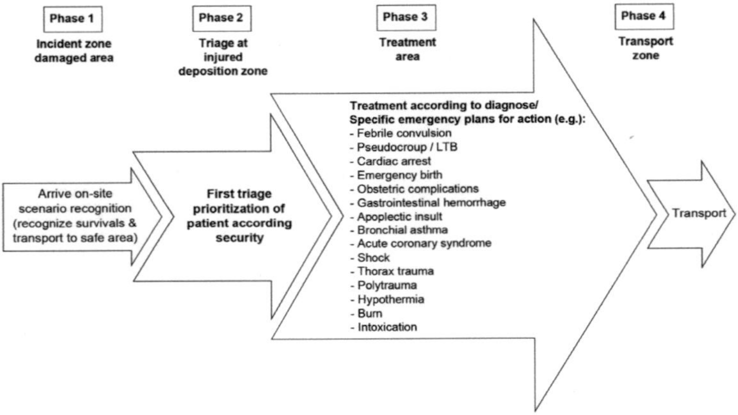

Figure 2.2: Rescue phases at MCI [PRS07]

Depending on the diagnosis and emergency of each patient, basic medical protocols and procedures are applied, for example, first or intensive cares, O2-provision with particular air flow, basic monitoring, and intravenous support. Subsequently, special care is provided including the provision of medicines, crystalloid solutions or especial emergency antidotes. Physicians only take decisions on the provision of special emergency medicaments.

This phase ends when the victim is prepared to be transported to a particular hospital, where it will receive special and individualized attention. The AIO performs the selection of the hospital and the organization of the transport.

Phase 4 - Transport

The transport planning depends on the emergency of the patient. This information is regularly controlled by the PED and informed to the MIO who coordinates, together with the AIO, the hospital selection.

The ambulance traffic area is prepared aside from the treatment area. There, all patient requiring transportation are dispatched. For the planning, some information aside from the diagnosis is required, such as the transport position (standing, sitting or lying). The PED also indicates the vehicle type. They are BLS ambulances for non-emergency patients, ALS vehicles for emergency patients, ALS vehicles with PED for emergency patients, ambulances with special pediatric equipment and emergency helicopters [Vem04].

2.1.2 Categorization and Prioritization of Patients

As described above, the tactical rescue plan and the efficient provision of medical assistance is only possible with the situational information of the incident, primordially based on the assessment, classification and prioritization of the patients. Only a PED can perform the categorization and prioritization process, and it is commonly called *Triage* [CM05, CFY02, KAGL96]

Triage: Definition and History

According to the Oxford English Dictionary the term triage comes from the French *trier*, that means *to sort* or *to cull*. Apparently, it was first applied to the sorting process of agricultural products, especially for the identification of broken coffee beans [Bla04, PD10]. Since the last century, this method has been adopted in emergency medicine to classify casualties according to the severity of injuries and the kind of illness. This classification establishes the need for care, the urgency and the place of treatment [Gon13].

Medical triage was first applied during the Napoleon's campaigns. The physician Dominique-Jean Larrey developed the concept, who, after joining the Army of Rhine, implemented a method to provide surgical care on-site. It was until after the battle of Waterloo, when he became Chief Surgeon of the Napoleonic Guard and Inspector General of the Office of Health of the Army. Later he became Chief Surgeon of the Royal Guard and a member of the Academy of Medicine and the Council of Health [SLZ+06, Mit08, Pea05, Sid12].

During his actions on the battlefield, Larrey was overloaded by the ad hoc, haphazard and unorganized treatment of battle casualties. It was there where his concern to prevent the wastage of medical resources grew. Larrey's work legacy is to the military medicine, who identified the necessity to sort the casualties, to manage better the medical resources in a scarcity scenario [KAGL96]. As Blagg et al. reports in [Bla04], that the memories of Dominique-Jena Larrey reflects for the first time in [LM32] the mass casualty problem and the triage objectives. The scenario is specially documented [LH14] in the memories of the Russian campaign:

> *„I had scarcely made the necessary preparations, when the wounded arrived in a crowd, and much confusion would have ensued, had I not pursued the order of dressing and arrangement, observed by me in all battles" ... „Those who are dangerously wounded must be tended first, entirely without regard to rank or distinction. Those less severely injured must wait until the gravely wounded have been operated on and dressed. The slightly wounded may go to the hospital line; specially officers, since they have horses and therefore have transport, and regardless, most of these have but trivial wounds".*

Modern Triage for Mass Casualty Incidents

Since the middle of the last century, emergency services and organizations have been evolved. As well, a dozen of triage-mechanisms has been conceived by different emergency and rescue organizations around the world. Their mission is to have a standard criteria to categorize the patients and to minimize the morbidity of the affected people maximizing the use of resources, even the condition of scarcity. Typically, the time to assess the patient varies from two to five minutes [PD10].

After ensuring a safe environment at the incident area, the EMS physicians are ready to perform the triage procedures. The process includes various assessment activities to determine the urgency of the patient. Triage is a very complex and can be easily influenced by the preparation and experience of the physician realizing the triage, the available resources, the age of the patient and the selected triage algorithm [LSC+08].

The execution of the triage requires ethical considerations; all patients should be assisted without any discrimination. Thus, it can only be applied by experienced and trained PEDs, which can perform the categorization by the defined protocols [Lee10]. Most of the modern MCI triage algorithms or protocols sort the treatment priority of the casualty into four-five basic categories. The classification depends on the severity of diseases or injuries:*immediate, delayed, minimal and expectant or death* [PD10].

Immediate medical assistance

This group stands for the patients with the highest priority and it is assigned to those with severe injuries that have the possibility to survive, receiving attention immediately. They might require first aid techniques, as hemorrhage control and airway support, before transportation to the healthcare facility for specialized assistance. Patients with breathing and circulation threats or in shock belong to this category.

Delayed medical assistance

Patients with sustained significant injuries may be categorized as delayed, for example, patients with internal or major fractures. They might require transportation, and medical assistance can wait until hospitalization occurs. However, they should be periodically supervised to avoid deterioration of their condition.

Minimal medical assistance

This category is commonly assigned to the walking wounded ones, and the ones that have minor and controllable injuries. These patients are stable and may not require hospitalization. Injuries are manageable by the paramedics on-site. Examples of these injuries are external and soft-tissue injuries, easy fractures or minor bleeding.

Expectant or death

Expectant victims have major injuries that even with the application of a considerable amount of medical resources and paramedics efforts the recovery probability remains low. The expenditure of medical assistance to these victims may compromise the clinical progress of those with a clear chance to survive. Some triage methodologies differentiate the expectant casualties from the death ones, assigning different categories. Expectant casualties only require palliative care. The assignation of this category involves ethical considerations. Thus, only an experienced physician can assign this group or declare the clinical death.

Patient triage is a dynamic process. In order to follow the progress of its medical condition, each patient should be assessed and categorized periodically. Thus, there is not a unique triage area; it can happen at the site where the accident occurred or in the treatment area. Accordingly to findings in rescue medicine literature, some of the most applied triage procedures are:

- *Simple Triage And Rapid Treatment (START)*
- *Modified Simple Triage And Rapid Treatment*
- *JumpSTART Pediatric Triage Algorithm*
- *SALT Mass Casualty Triage Algorithm (Sort, Assess, Lifesaving, Interventions, Treatment/Transport)*
- *Triage Sieve*
- *CareFlight Triage*

START, m-START and JumpSTART

In 1983, the Newport Beach Fire and Marine Department and Hoag Hospital in California developed the Simple Triage and Rapid Treatment. Since then, it has remained as the most popular triage algorithm, at least in US and Germany. Initially, it assessed the ability to obey commands; it observed the respiratory rate and the radial pulse, to determine the urgency category [SGB+06, CM05]. Figure 2.3(b) shows the algorithm m-START.

The START algorithm has evolved into new versions where instead of considering the capillary refill, it evaluates the radial pulse. In recent modifications, it also takes into account the ability to walk.

JumpSTART is the most commonly applied pediatric triage among the EMS during MCI. Aside the victim classification and prioritization, it looks forward to reducing the emotional burden of the PED. In 1995 at the Miami, Florida Hospital for Children by Dr. Lou Romig conceived the children version [Rom11]. It is an adaptation of the START adult triage algorithm for the categorization of pediatric casualties.

SALT

The endorsement of Sort-Asses-Lifesaving Interventions-Treatment and Transport algorithm is an effort of different American associations of PEDs. The well-known American College of Emergency Physicians participated to provide a standardize all-hazards MCI triage for all casualties, including adults and children. SALT is primordially divided in two steps: a global sorting and an individualized assessment [Lee10, LSC+08].

Firstly, the global sorting occurs, prioritizing the patients for an individual and deeper assessment. Those, who can walk are assigned with the lowest priority, followed by those who can at least obey commands or wave their limbs. The patients who do not move and who have an apparent life-threatening condition receive the highest priority and should be assessed first in the second step.

The second assessment begins with lifesaving interventions, e.g., hemorrhage control, airway support, chest decompression and provision of medicaments. Then, the patients are prioritized for a correct distribution of treatment and transport, optimizing the application of resources. With this aim, PED classifies the victims in one of the five categories already mentioned, see Figure 2.3(d).

Triage Sieve and Pediatric Triage Tape

Both triage algorithms are a very similar to START and Jump- START. They are widely used throughout the UK, Sweden, India, Australia, South Africa, and they are also an accepted method for military use in the North Atlantic Treaty Organization (NATO).

Originally, Triage Sieve stratified patients based on the patient's walking capacity and the breath and heart rate (HR). Lately, the heart rate was replaced by the capillary refill. In contrast to the START algorithm, Triage Sieve does not assess the consciousness of the patient. Triage Sieve categorizes the patients in four priority classes: urgent, immediate, delayed and dead [HHMS98, NG99a, RAV^{+}10], as Figure 2.3(a).

The pediatric triage is presented on a waterproof tape with information that relates the height and age of the patient to the acceptable range of the physiological parameters. It just needs to be placed aside and parallel to the child, determining the weight and age of the child based on its height. Figure 2.4 shows this calibration tape.

CareFlight

CareFlight triage algorithm was developed in North Wales, Australia. This triage algorithm evaluates, similar to START, the ability to obey commands, the respiration and the radial pulse. In contrast to the START algorithm, it does not assess the breath rate and the mental status is tested in the first place.

Figure 2.3(c) shows the algorithm. CareFlight triage algorithm assesses qualitatively the patient's condition. Thus, it is considered a fast assessment technique, but it has the disadvantage to oversee some isolated breathing complications [NG99b, GLHS01, Gar03] .

Despite several attempts to demonstrate which triage method is the most accurate; there is no consistency in the results reported by different journals on EMS. Due to its popularity and common use, this dissertation refers to modified START as a triage algorithm.

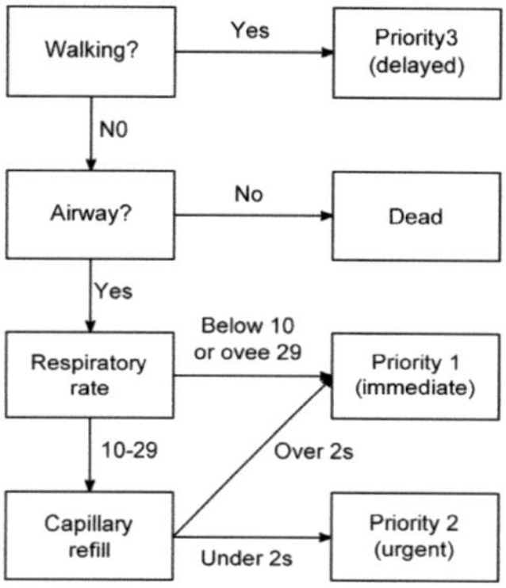

(a) Triage Sieve

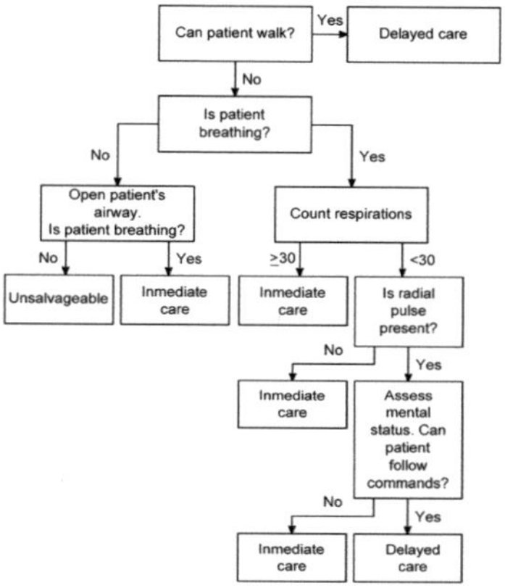

(b) Modified Simple Triage and Rapid Treatment

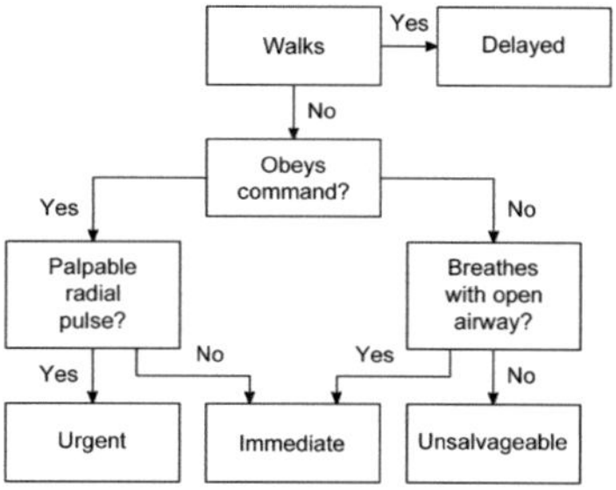

(c) CareFlight Triage

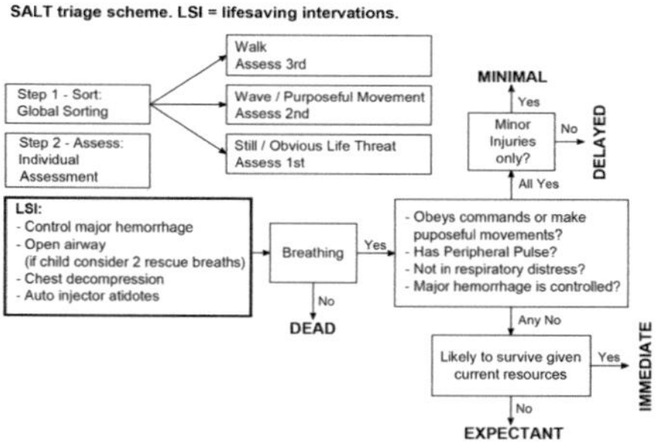

(d) SALT Triage

Figure 2.3: Different algorithms for the triage of victims during MCI scenarios [BKS96][Lee10]

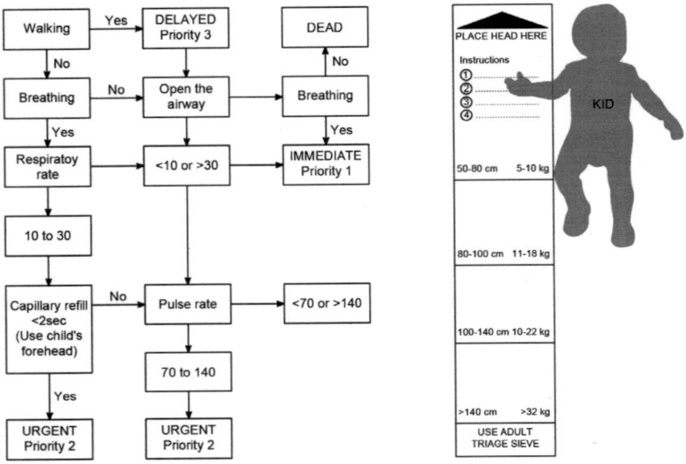

Figure 2.4: Pediatric Triage Tape [LKG+11]

2.1.3 On-site Information and Communication Systems

On MCI, scenarios triage information is vital for a successful tactical planning. As mentioned before, it helps to prioritize the access to the medical assistance and the transportation of the patients. The triage is performed on-site by the PEDs, and the resultant category should be informed to the incident commander. The triage information should also be available and visible on the field with the objective to be a reference and to guide the care actions of the paramedics.

Different support communication and information systems have been already implemented to support the rescue logistics within the incident area. Triage tags have been adapted to protocol and to show information right on the field. These are distributed to all casualties and consist typically of a paper card protected by a plastic bag and a cord to attach it to the victim. There, the PED documents its assessment and interventions. He also writes down the personal information of the patients, identifies locations of injuries and illness, vital signs, select the type of transport and ongoing treatments, such as intravenous fluids and medicaments [Gar03] [KWF12].

Table 2.1: Triage categories, color code and decision criteria

Category	Color Code	Decision Criteria
I: Immediate	Red	spontaneous breathing after reanimation respiratory rate higher than 30 pulse absent capillary refill higher than 2 sec does not obey commands
II:Delayed	Yellow	breathing rate lower than 30 pulse present capillary refill lower than 2 sec obeys commands
III: Minor	Green	able to walk
IV: Expectant	**Black**	no breathing

Aside this information, a PED declares the triage category by selecting a colored card. Herewith, it is possible to identify from a certain distance the status of the casualties. A plenty of triage card models exist, but the color code among the different tags and algorithms is the same [HCP08] [PD10]. Table 2.1 relates the triage color code and categories. Figure 2.5(a) explains the decision-making process to determine patient's priority according to the START algorithm. categories and conditions for each color. Figure 2.5(b) presents the mentioned triage cards.

The protocoled on-tag information needs to be passed to the organization commander and the MIO. Written documentation and horizontal voice direct communication are the ordinary means to pass the information on the field. After physicians categorized the victims and filled out the triage tag, paramedics on the field collect the same data from the triage tags on worksheet [MW12]. Paramedics give in hand the information to the organization commander, or they use peer to peer communication such as walkie-talkies [CARQ01].

The MIO has to gather and to interpret the information. A magnetic board is used by the commanders to organize the information, as the boards shown in Figure 2.6. Aside the triage information, the IMO organizes information, such as availability of medical resources, transport already on-site, a general position of resource, available medical personnel among others.

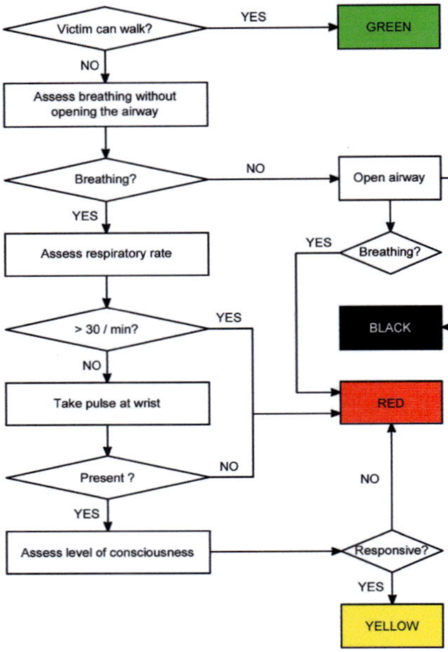

(a) START algorithm

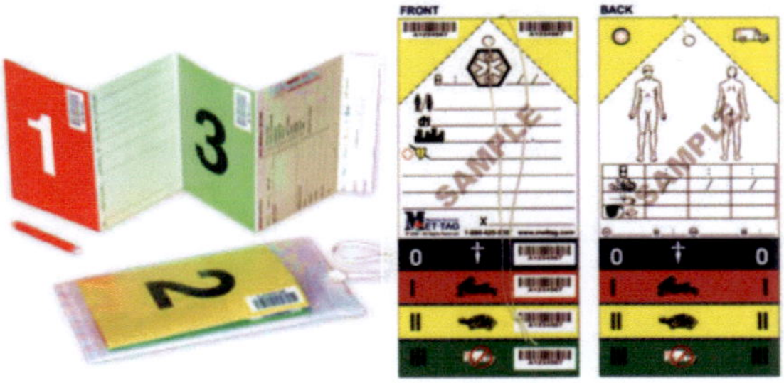

(b) Triage paper cards

Figure 2.5: Triage START algorithm and paper triage cards[RHG+14]

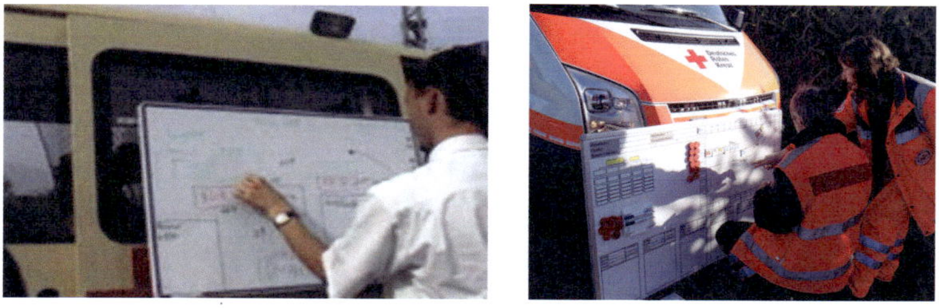

(a) (b)

Figure 2.6: Rescue planning whiteboards for incident officers [CS09]

MCI is a very dynamic scenario that requires an intense collection of standardized information and communication process. Re-triage and re-evaluation should be continuously performed; this to acquire a more accurate snapshot of the situation [RAV^{+}10] . Despite the efforts to standardize nationally and internationally the information systems and communication methods, there is a variety of methods and systems applied among the emergency and relief agencies. This diversity complicates the operations that involve rescue forces from different nations, and even from different districts in the same country, [NG99b] [AF12].

2.2 Physiology of the Trauma Casualty

As mentioned, MCI scenarios are the result of an unexpected and radical change of the commonness in a very short period, affecting the surround of a considerable number of persons. This scenario can only be possible with the expenditure of an enormous amount of uncontrolled energy. This violent release of energy, when persons are at the incident area, produces on them different types of injuries and wounds; besides the possible compromise of their vital functions.

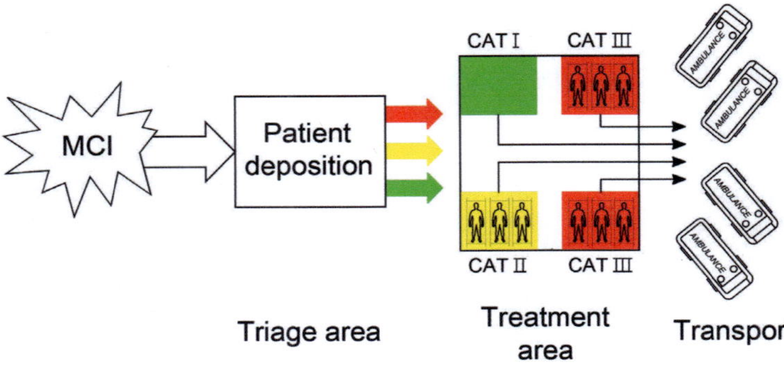

Figure 2.7: Triage, treatment and transport areas

Trauma is the medical term for the injuries or illness produced in an accident or by an external medium. Emergency medicine and traumatology are the fields of the medicine to attend the clinical problems derived from the injury. Injuries can affect any corporal zone, affecting any of the physiologic system [?]. For this reason, PEDs are formed in diverse specialties and provide care to any victim. Typical relief tasks are to suture severe lacerations, attend fractures and dislocations, manage a heart attack and respiration damage, stop hemorrhages, and to support shock and hysteria. The main purpose of the physician is to stabilize and to maintain the vital functions of the casualty, in the way it can continue receiving a more personalized assistance at the health care center.

2.2.1 The Golden Hour of Trauma

Time is the most important constraint after an incident occurred, and it is a challenge to be defeated by the trauma and emergency medicine. The time between the incident and the attention defines the survival chances, as the life expectancy and quality of recovery.

In the 1970s, trauma centers started to be seriously developed. Before, the emergency care consisted in the scoop-and-run approach, no care or very little care was provided during transport to the next facility. In 1974, after a personal and familiar incident, Dr. James Styner, recognized the necessity to provide medical assistance at the event place and during transportation. He realized that even the local health care facilities were not able to provide better support care than on the field with reduced resources [RYS+12, CK10].

From his point of view, this new approach for the management of the injuries on the field would reduce the morbidity when applying essential medical assistance. This approach set a reference to the urgent need of medical care of a trauma patient, also named as the *golden hour of trauma* [LSC+08]. It starts with the incident and not with the first contact with the victim. The golden hour of trauma gives a reference to the survival chances of the casualty. It depends notably on the type and severity of the injury. Clark JR et al. present a study of the time to operation for patients with abdominal injuries, establishing a reduction rate in the survival probability of one percent every three minutes. After one hour, the survival probability for this kind of injuries is about 45% [CTD+02], see Figure 2.8.

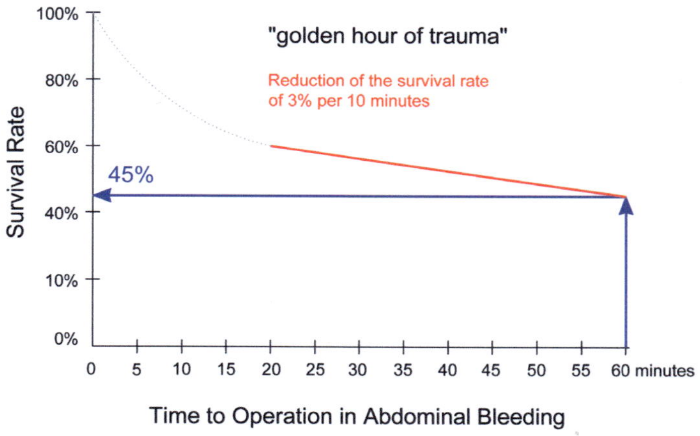

Figure 2.8: The golden hour of trauma, as in [CTD+02]

During disaster management, prioritization of casualties is a requirement to arrange medical provision. Benson et al. provide in [BKS96] a graph estimating the probability to reduce mortality after administering medical assistance on the different type of victims, see Figure 2.9. It takes into consideration the benefit of providing medical care, the survival proba-bility and the cost in resources. Resources include physicians, parame-dics, time applying care and supplies.

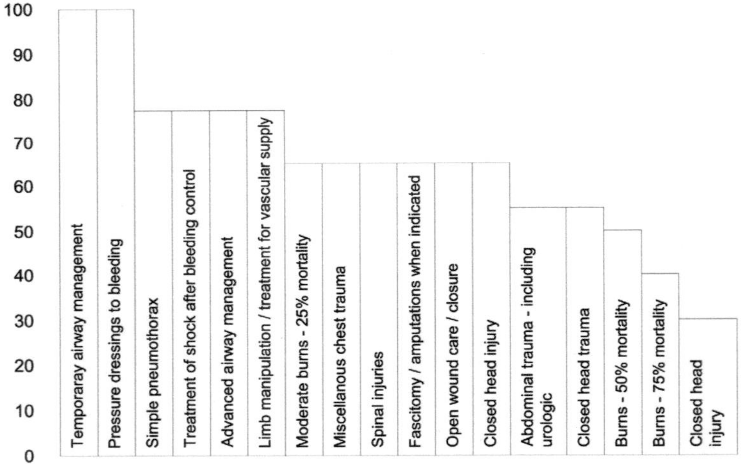

Figure 2.9: Treatment priority depending on medical care and injury [BKS96]

2.2.2 Injuries, Wounds and Assessment

Among the most common injuries are crushed limbs, head injury, chest and abdominal trauma, burns and spinal trauma. Figure 2.10 reflects injury mechanism in two typical accident scenarios. This processes can be transferred to other incident scenarios. After identifying the priority of the casualty, they are managed in the treatment area. While waiting for transport, each patient is treated depending on the injury and illness type [CK10].

Aside the triage information, which works as a tactical reference, the PED documents the diagnosis and evaluates the injuries individually. This information will indicate the paramedics the maneuver to assist the injuries and keep the casualty stable.

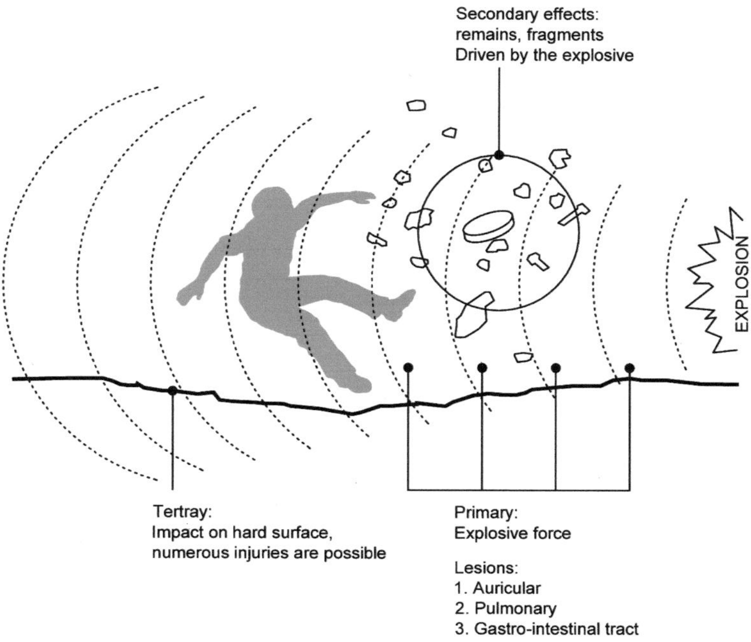

Figure 2.10: Examples of wound causes [CK10]

Benson et al. present also in [BKS96] different scores have been developed to treat specific emergencies, for example:

MESS - Mangled Extremity Severity Score

Crunched limbs may be a common problem during MCI. They challenge the physicians and paramedics to decide which extremity attempt to salvage and which to amputate. In order to support this difficult decision, the mangled extremity severity score (MESS) can be applied. The score evaluates the tissue disruption and the compromise of the circulation condition. Other parameters like the age and signs of shock and blood pressure are taken into consideration.

Glasgow Comma Scale

The Glasgow coma scale is the reference for a neurologic assessment. It is applied as a reference for the evaluation of the mental status of the casualty. It distinguishes between different ranges of conditions, going from good to severe disable. It gives an orientation to possible vegetative state or death, and it is also a reference to the chance to survive with or without a mental disability. It is based on the assessment of eye-opening and motor and verbal response.

An accurate assessment and treatment should only proceed in a clinic with unlimited resources. While, on the emergency field, the treatment is reduced to the protection of the brain oxygen-supply and the head elevation. If possible and required, burr holes are done, for example in patients with dilated pupils.

In the cases of burns, which are also a typical trauma during MCI, evaluation and treatments depend fundamentally on the age, body region and the amount of the damaged area. Survival chances are greater between the ages of 15 and 30 years. Medical assistance to casualties with burns requires an intense application of resources. Thus, resuscitation and further treatment should be evaluated carefully under austere conditions.

Chest injuries and abdominal trauma require the constant assessment of vital signs. Chest and abdomen are the zones that contain and protect the organs performing the physiological functions. Thus, these victims require continuous monitoring and in the case of severe injuries, patients will require urgent attention and transport. Casualties with internal injuries and without an evident wound are a primary concern for the paramedics. These casualties may be able to walk and under categorized since these patients can suddenly suffer a shock. A regular control of the vital signs may help to distinguish better these cases [Ina11a].

2.2.3 Physiological Systems and Functions

The primary task of emergency health workers is to keep casualties stable before they can receive specialized medical attention. The severity of the injury indicates the priority to receive medical care depending on how much life supporting functions have been affected. Different systems perform life-supporting functions which are in charge to provide nutrients and oxygen to all the cells of the subsystems, organs and tissues of the body, as well to collect all the wastage. The systems in charge to perform the vital functions are the respiratory and circulatory systems, they are regulated through the neural system [CK10] [GAR+05] [GAR+07].

Respiratory System

The respiratory system is in charge of the ventilation. It supports the particle exchange of oxygen O2 and carbon dioxide CO2 between the external environment and the body. O2 is vital for the cells to perform their functions. Chemical reactions in the cells liberate energy and CO2, which needs to be expelled from the body. This particles exchange happens in the alveoli that are guarded by the lungs [GAR+05].

The respiratory system is formed by the upper airways, conformed by the nose and mouth, passing through the throat and trachea until the lungs. Before the trachea reaches the lungs, it is divided into two branches. These branches are known as primary bronchi, which are again subdivided into the second and third branches, the last branch is the bronchiole, and at the end of the bronchiole, the alveoli are found. The exchange of particles with the blood takes place in the alveoli. The red globules are responsible for transporting the O2 and CO2 in the blood.

The ventilation is the result of the mechanic expansion and contraction of the diaphragm, which at the same time produce the contraction and expansion of the lungs. The contraction produces the exhalation and the increase the inhalation. This action, known as breathing, is usually regulated autonomously by the parasympathetic system, but it can occur consciously. For example, this helps to stop breathing under the water.

Circulatory System

The circulatory system is responsible for transporting the nutrients, substances and particles necessary for the well-function of the cells of all organs and tissues. The principal actor in the circulatory system is the heart, which pumps the blood through arteries, vessels and veins. The heart is connected to two circuits of arteries and veins, one for the transport of blood to all the body and the other to support the exchange of O2 and CO2 at the alveoli [GAR+05, Web09].

The heart is a four-hollow organ, formed by two auricles and two ventricles. Auricles and ventricles on each side are only separated by the cuspidal and tricuspid valve. Auricles are only a pre-chamber, which stores the blood whereas the main pumping action are executed by the ventricles. In the relaxation phase, known as diastole, blood flows from the auricles to the ventricles. During a contraction, known as systole, the valves are closed, and blood is pumped to the body through and to the lungs. Blood flows back to heart through.

An electrical pulse, generate at the node, commands the heart-pumping action. This pulse flows through the heart tissue producing the contraction of the ventricles. The heart activity is regulated mainly by the parasympathetic system.

Sympathetic and Parasympathetic Functions

The nervous system controls and regulates a vast of physical and physiological functions. A central and peripheral systems perform the whole neural activity. The central system, formed by the brain and the spinal cord; and a peripheral system, formed by a network of nerves connecting all organs and tissues to the brain. Receptors around the body generate messages in the form of an electrical pulse, which are continuously processed by the neurons that conform the brain structure. Depending on the function, different regions of the brain react generating an answer to the received messages. [GAR+05, Web09].

The brain regulates both unconscious and conscious corporal functions and activities. Life support functions like the heart action or the unconscious breathing or functions of the digestive organs are controlled automatically by the parasympathetic system. Motor function and verbal communication are regulated by the sympathetic system. Thus, a threat to the nervous system produced by a head or spinal injury, also produces a damage to the physiological systems.

2.3 Ambulant and Noninvasive Physiological Assessment

The tactical planning, as well as the treatment procedures, requires a continuous assessment of the physiological and vital functions of the casualty. In the last sections, it has been mentioned that the circulatory and respiratory systems are the life-functions supporting system. Different tools and methods are applied by the physicians and paramedics for the assessment and monitoring of these both systems.

Due to the urgency to prioritize the casualties, the assessment methods to proceed with the triage algorithms are merely manual, whereas in the treatment area and during transportation, new and sophisticated technologies are used. Various parameters serve as a reference for the condition of both systems, e.g. the heart rate and the breath rate. Different techniques and instruments for their assessment are described in this section.

2.3.1 Assessment of the Circulatory System

The heart action commands the vascular or circulatory system. The heart contraction is regulated by a rhythmic electrical pulse. This rhythm is a result of a vast number of factors such as age, gender, emotions, corporal activity, illness, etc., and it is an indication of the well function of the heart.

The mechanical work of the heart produces a blood torrent, whose force has one vectorial component in the direction of the vessels producing a flow, and another force component acting on the wall of the vessels. The assessment of this effect in an individual area is known as blood pressure, and it is also a reference of the well function of the heart. The pressure during the maximum heart contraction is known as systolic pressure, while, during maximum relaxation, it is known as diastolic, and both can indicate different malfunctions.

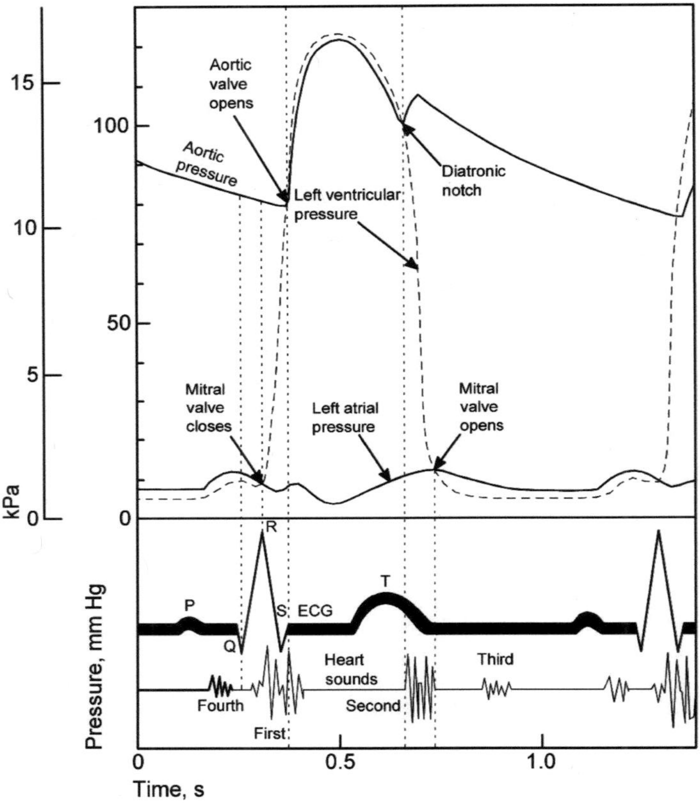

Figure 2.11: Measurable signals from the heart action [Web09]

The electrical and mechanical action, as well as the rhythm of the heart, gives a reference of its condition. These actions produce different parameters that are measurable. Some of the techniques applied during urgencies to assess the circulatory condition of the casualties are explained here:

Manual Assessment

The manual assessment allows a rapid technique, which is important under urgent and austere conditions. Only the mechanical action of the heart is possible to be assessed manually. It produces an effect against the wall; that is palpable at different body regions, such as the limbs and throat, where considerably big vessels are passing through. This tangible effect is known as the radial pulse [GAR+05]

Another measurable parameter is the refill of the finger veins, which is an indicator of a good irrigation, a result of enough blood pressure. The assessment proceeds by pressing the nail of a finger and controlling the time that takes to recover the red tone under the nail [SHS+11, GLHS01].

The mechanical cardiac activity produces a tone. Fig. 2.11 indicates the sound produced by the cardiac activity. This tone is auscultated with a stethoscope. The sound also gives a reference to the performance and some pathologies of the hollowed cardiac organ. The heart rate can be determined when the rhythm of sound or radial pulse is measured against a time reference [Web09].

On-site Medical Instrumentation - Electrocardiogram (ECG)

The electrical pulse of the heart is only assessable with sophisticated medical instrumentation. The electrical pulse is originated by the natural pacemaker sinoatrial (SA) node, located between the right auricle and the superior vena cava. The originated pulse reaches through three electrical pathways (anterior, middle and posterior tracts) the atrioventricular (AV) nodes. There, the pulse is delayed until it continues through the bundle of His and reaches the ventricle cells following a complicated electrical pathway [Web09].

The ventricle cells are surrounded by a plasma membrane, which allows the contact with the next cell so that the electrical pulse is transmitted from cell to cell. They form the *myofibrils* conforming the cardiac tissue at the ventricles. This fiber is contractile, and it is responsible for contraction of both ventricles in the presence of an electric pulse.

The heart works as an electric dipole with variable magnitude and orientation, which generates different current strengths that flow through the thorax and reach the body surface. Potential measured at the skin surface is known as *electrocardiogram (ECG)*. The ECG is formed by the P wave, the QRS complex, and the T wave. The first wave is produced by the auricles depolarization; the complex is produced by the ventricular depolarization and the last wave results of the ventricular polarization (see Fig. 2.12).

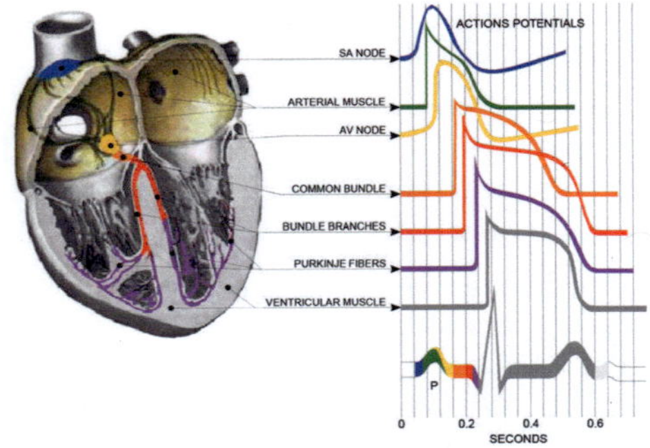

Figure 2.12: Electrocardiogram generation [Web09]

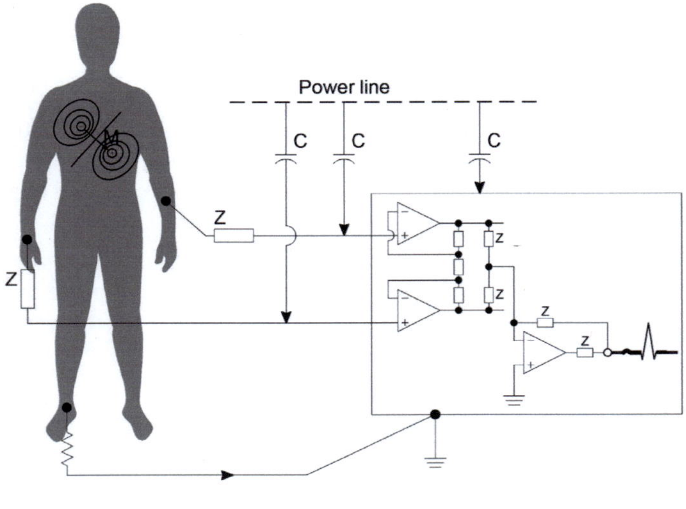

Figure 2.13: Electrocardiograph [Web09]

Potential on the surface of the skin can be acquired by placing a pair of electrodes at predefined locations, defined by the limbs. A pair of electrodes placed at different positions yields different potentials. This pair of electrodes is referred as lead. Normally the lead I is monitored, and it is obtained placing the electrodes taking as reference the superior limbs. The potential is filtered, for the sake of noise reduction and amplified to obverse the ECG. HR and specific cardiac conditions can be identified by the assessment of the EGC. Portable electrocardiographs are commonly used by paramedics (see Figure 2.13) [GAR+05].

On-site Medical Instrumentation - Sphygomanometer

Assessment of blood pressure is a standard clinical procedure. The best method to measure blood pressure is invasive, and it is done with the introduction of a catheter where a direct monitoring of the blood pressure is possible. However, this requires special skills and instrumentation, which is not practicable during rescue operations.

An indirect and noninvasive method is also possible and more suitable for the assessment of casualties. It consists of the palpation or the sound detection of the pulse distal to an occlusive cuff. Figure 2.14 depicts a sphygmomanometer, which consists of an inflatable cuff for vessel occlusion, a bulb to inflate the cuff and a mercury or aneroid manometer which indicates the pressure [Web09].

The cuff is inflated pressing the vessel above the systolic pressure. Then, the cuff is slowly bled off, reducing its pressure gradually. When the pressure in the cuff is lower than the systolic pressure, blood start to spurts and radial pulse is then palpable while placing a stethoscope over the artery, the first Korotkoff sound is detectable. At that instant the manometer indicates the systolic pressure, when the cuff pressure is lower than the diastolic pressure, the Korotkoff is not more audible, and the manometer shows the diastolic pressure. Modern instrumentation allows an automatic indirect blood pressure.

2.3.2 Assessment of the Respiratory System

The breathing activity relies on the mechanical expansion and contraction of the lungs. This action satisfies the air renewal required for the gas exchange at the alveoli, through the inhalation and exhalation. Different parameters are indicators of the integrity of the respiratory system, such as the air flow, the rhythmic contraction and expansion of the thorax, which are direct indicators of the integrity of the respiratory system. Other parameters, like the air volume and the oxygen saturation, are also indicators of the well-function of the respiratory system, but they are not directly observable, a special medical instrumentation is required. The measurement of air flow with devices that require intubation are not recommended on the field or during transportation unless both are integrated. Otherwise, they can interfere with other care maneuvers [RR92].

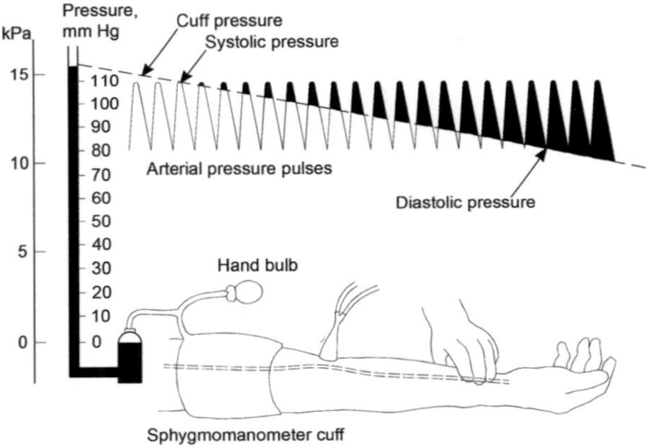

Figure 2.14: Principle of sphygmomanometer [Web09]

Manual Assessment

A direct and manual assessment of the respiratory condition is possible. This assessment supports the prioritization the casualties during an urgent scenario. The breathing is assessable visually, tactilely and audibly. A regular breathing will be identified by three methods. The visual assessment consists in the evaluation of the skin tone; a blue tone will indicate hypoxia. The rhythmical contraction and expansion of the thorax is also visible and palpable, however, in some cases it might be difficult to assess. An acute evaluation will result from the identification of warm air coming off from the upper airways [GAR^{+}05].

A more reliable assessment method will be the auscultation of the air flow with a stethoscope; breathing noise provides information of different problems and pathologies along the respiratory system.

On-site Medical Instrumentation - Pulse Oximetry (SpO2)

The objective of the respiratory system is to provide the blood with enough oxygen and to clean it from dioxide carbon. An assessment of the oxygen level in the blood will be an indirect indicator that the respiratory system is accomplishing its task integrally. Low oxygen levels in the blood will be an indicator of multiple pathologies, going from the obstruction of the airway to more complex problem, which are not identified manually [Web09, BU12].

A noninvasive method to evaluate the oxygen saturation in the blood is known as pulse oximetry . It is based on the concept of the photoplethysmograph. It measures the light modulation resulting from a change in blood volume produced by the pulse wave in the vessels. This measurement is performed in thick regions, where the light can reach the arteries, as in the earlobes, fingers, lips and toes [Web09].

The measurement principle relies on the influence of the oxygen on the color of the hemoglobin (Hb). Oxygen saturated hemoglobin (HbO2) is red, whereas Hb has a blue tone. This difference has an impact on the light absorption of the blood. Light is radiated through the tissues and vessels, a portion of the light, the not absorbed part, is detected by a photodetector placed on the skin surface [BU12], see Figure 2.15(a).

The absorption factor is defined as follows:

$$\alpha = \sum_{\mu} \varepsilon_{\mu} (\lambda)\, c_{\mu} \tag{2.1}$$

Where α is the absorption coefficient which depends on the wavelength λ of the light source. The molar extinction coefficient ε is specific for each substance, it differs between Hb02 and Hb, μ indicates the index for each substance, and c defines the concentration of Hb or HbO2.

The external photodetector absorbs the rest of the light, depends on the wavelength (lambda) and the light intensity of the source, the substance and the width of the medium. As more than one substance composes the blood, the light absorption will depend on the concentration of each substance present in the blood. In pulse oximetry, the calculation of HbO2% is under consideration and requires two light sources with two different wavelengths for the distinction between HbO2 and Hb.

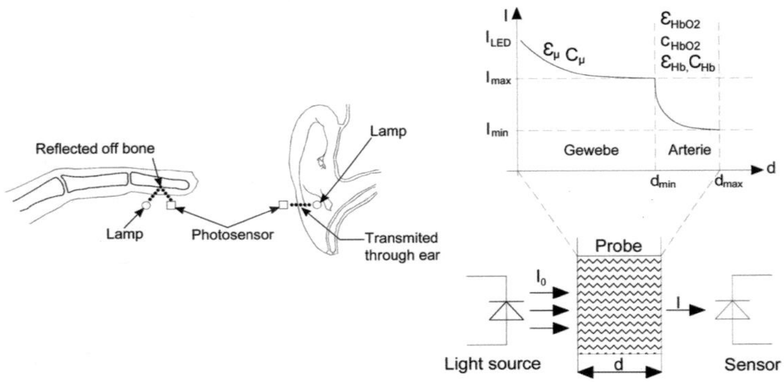

(a) Main routine algorithm

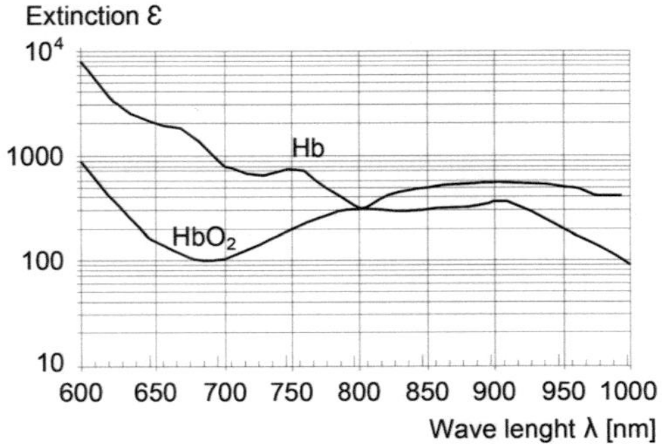

(b) Interrupt architecture cards

Figure 2.15: Principles of pulse oximetry [BU12, Web09]

Typically red light ($\lambda 1 = 660nm$) and infrared light ($\lambda 2 = 920nm$) are selected. By $\lambda 1$, Hb dominates the light absorption, HbO2 does it by $\lambda 2$. This difference is the base to calculate the concentration of HbO2. In Figure 2.15(b) the absorption spectrum for Hb and HbO2 is depicted. Oxygen saturation is presented as the ratio of HbO2 in the blood (HbO2 + Hb) [BU12, CU05].

The medium is formed by different tissues and bone, only the light absorption in the blood is under consideration. The pulse action of the heart would produce a distance variation between the source and the sensor, also varying the concentration of the substance and the absorption coefficient, see Figure 2.15. At the diastole, the photodetector produces $Imax$ at the systole $Imin$. The current is reduced exponentially by α and the width of the measurement probe d:

$$I_{max} = I\left(\lambda, d_{diastole}\right) = I_{LED} \cdot e^{-\alpha(\lambda) \cdot d_{diastole}} \tag{2.2}$$

$$I_{min} = I\left(\lambda, d_{systole}\right) = I_{LED} \cdot e^{-\alpha(\lambda) \cdot d_{systole}} \tag{2.3}$$

The absorption coefficients for Hb and HbO2 are calculated as follows:

$$\alpha_{Hb} = ln \frac{Imin\left(\lambda_1\right)}{Imax\left(\lambda_1\right)} \tag{2.4}$$

$$\alpha_{HbO2} = ln \frac{Imin\left(\lambda_2\right)}{Imax\left(\lambda_2\right)} \tag{2.5}$$

The relation between α_{Hb} and α_{HbO2} provides a reference to estimate the oxygen saturation in the blood.

The photodetector will generate a current that, with a trans-impedance amplifier, is transduced into a potential that is filtered and amplified, resulting in an electrical signal called *pleth curve*. The pleth curve is a result of a cardiac pulse; hereby the estimation of heart rate is also possible [CU05].

Another characteristic of the pleth curve is the perfusion index (PI). The PI indicate the strength of the pulse and normally is calculated from the curved resulted from infrared light modulation. It expresses the ratio between the pulsatile and non-pulsatile components of the pleth curve. PI values are in the range from 0.2% to 20%, low values would be an indication of health problems. Values under 1.4% are related to higher morbidity and mortality. PI is affected by the monitoring conditions [LB05].

Portable pulse oximeter is common for the assessment of casualties, figure 2.16 presents one example of this device used on the field.

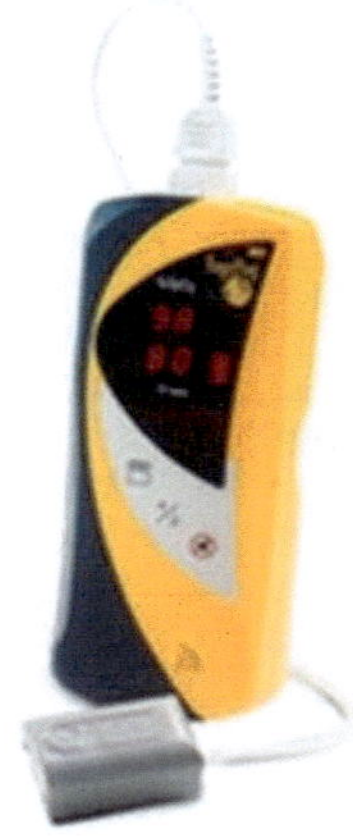

Figure 2.16: BCI 3401 Fingerprint Pulse Oximeter with Printer, 167 x 70 x 36mm (www.gpsupplies.com)

2.4 Summary

Several aspects of MCI scenarios are discussed. The rescue process during MCI is explained in detail. The role that incident commanders and officers play in the organization of the rescue logistic is described. Incident officers have to find out as soon as possible, which patient, needs what and which one need it first. For this purpose, the term triage is introduced. It is explained that the rescue plan relies on the triage information. Different triage methods and tools are introduced. The ordinary tools, as triage paper cards and whiteboards, are as well explained.

Typical patient conditions are described together with the physiological systems that are normally affected. Different tools to support the assessment of patients at emergency scenarios are presented.

Next chapter discusses how different research groups have attempted to introduce new information and communication technologies (ICT) to support the triage and documentation process. The objective is to support the tactical planning of the first response accelerating the communication on the field.

3 Information and Communication Systems for MCI

Triage information is crucial for the clearance of the incident scenario, as well for the provision of adequate medical assistance. Medical care and transport to health care facilities are organized according to the priority of the casualty physiological state. Time is a major concern for the trauma and emergency medicine. Casualty's condition should continuously be monitored and evaluated to optimize the medical resources on the field. In this chapter, the state of the art and new ICT advances for the documentation of medical and tactical information during MCI are discussed.

In the last chapter, the triage term, methods and tools, as the triage tag, were introduced. The triage tag is the core tool for the documentation of medical and tactical information about the casualty on the field. However, the nature of the tag requires a considerable amount of manual effort to collect and document the relevant information it retains. The management of the triage tag information can result in a very tedious and time-consuming process; being not adequate for MCI situations.

New advances in ICTs represent a possibility for the improvement of the information management at MCI scenarios. Different research groups around the globe have seen on new technologies a chance to support the rescue management logistics and to accelerate the communication process. During the last decade a dozen of new platforms has been developed and studied, including satellite communication cells, autonomous wireless sensors and different sensor-based approaches for the automatic and remote monitoring of casualties. This chapter introduces and discusses some of the most relevant.

3.1 State of the Art

In Section 2.1.3 a brief overview of the information tools and communication methods was depicted. In this section, a profound analysis and critic of the state of the art is provided. Lessons learned from MCI and requirements to set new solutions gathering the last advances in ICTs are as well discussed.

The operation's logistic to clear the emergency scenario and to provide effectively medical care depends on the reliability of the available ICT. As before described, paper triage tags, paper protocols and direct voice communication, sometimes supported by walkie-talkies constitutes the ordinary information and communication tools during MCI scenarios.

The just above mentioned tools, when compared to the recent advances in ICT, appear to be rudimental. Lessons learned shows that actual means only represent either a solution for small scale MCI situations, up to 25 casualties or they serve only as documentation tools [VTEC86]. Different studies show that during massive rescue operations, the manual information management prolongs the communication process, threatening the time to attention and the time to transport of the casualties. Moreover, this situation increases the stress and frustration of paramedics and physicians. These and other lessons learned are discussed in this section.

3.1.1 The Paradigm of Triage Tag & its Disadvantages

The triage tags, when used, have been the most common tool to track and to document the patient priority and diagnose, as a treatment and transport maneuver on the field. Experienced emergency physician evaluate the patient physiological condition accordingly to the selected triage rules. This information is written manually on the tag, and it is the base for the organization of the rescue operation.

Multiple triage tags versions are available, but they consist primordially of a thin and hard plastic bag with colored cards. On the surface of the bag, physicians document by handwriting the casualty information (triage category, injured zones, illness, required treatment and transport, and personal information). Some of them guard a much more complex medical protocol, which the physicians also fulfill. This protocol provides a better diagnose of the patient supporting the individualized diagnose described, but it also requires more time to be fulfilled.

The nature of the triage tag constrains the rest of the information flow and communication process. The information on the card is relevant for the decision-making process during the whole operation. Therefore, it should be protocoled and continually reported to the commanders. This information has an impact on the provision of BLS and ALS and transport of the casualties. As well, communication technologies influence the on-site coordination between the health workers, and outside for the coordination between authorities, hospital and press. Figure 3.1 describes this information constitution at different phases of the rescue operation.

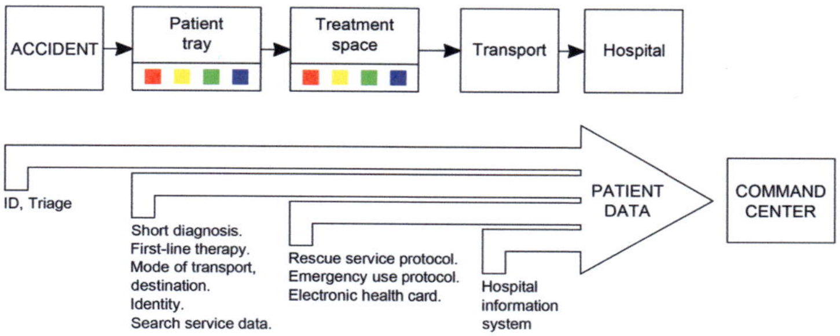

Figure 3.1: Information demand and flow during MCI [DAGM12]

The protocoling process involves a well manual handwriting documentation. Health workers supporting the organizational leader are randomly deployed around the casualties on the field to collect and organize the information from the tag on the organizational protocol. The triage data is later provided to the organizational commander and the senior emergency physician so they can count the patients according to the status priority, and estimate the need for medical and transportation resources.

The organizational leader receives the paper protocols in hand, or these are over voice communication reported. They track advances of the operation and set the rescue plan on a whiteboard. In the last chapter, figure 2.6 depicts different examples of organizational whiteboards for emergency scenarios. Following the communication and organizational chain, the information is relevant for the incident commander in order to coordinate with the corresponding authorities and hospital the need of resources.

As in section 2.2 explained; the physiology of the casualty is variant, and time-to-attention affected, therefore, casualties' triage should be evaluated and updated. As a result, the data collection and organization effort increases and depends on the number of victims and the disposability of physicians and health workers to perform the protocols.

In addition to the paperwork, during the triage other problems arise. For example, the lack of geographical information, which has to be also continually reported and matched with references at the incident site. Additionally most of the triage and treatment areas are outdoor sets. The weather conditions, especially the humidity and rain might treat the paper triage cards and paper protocols. Even the plastic protection bag, they have to be removed for documentation. Also, blood and other substances or visual obstacles might affect the visibility of the information.

In the theory, triage tags represent a logical and methodological solution to track and report patient data, and to support the MCI management, but in the practice they have failed. The triage tag, the paper protocol and the direct voice communication are not a reliable solution to help the logistic of a rescue operation. Moreover, they increase the challenge of the situation and disturbs the rescue organization; they do not provide accurate information because the times between triage and report are unknown.

The next section discusses punctual problems and difficulties of the state of the art of information systems and communication methods for MCI management.

3.1.2 Experiences with Triage Tags & Lessons Learned

This section discusses experiences and lessons learned about the use and application of triage tag and paper documentation. Also, multiple research organizations around the globe have been advocated to document and discuss such experiences. The results are not positive, and they encourage the necessity to improve the information systems and communications methods to promote a more efficient MCI management.

Problems with triage tag have been reported since the 80's. For example, Vayer et al. in their work *New Concepts in Triage*, 1986, analyzed experiences from 25 MCI situations, collected from *The Royal Victoria Hospital in Belfast* between 1969 and 1976 [VTEC86]. They point that possible failure reasons of the triage tags are unfamiliarity of the users, static information in a dynamic process; fulfillment requires time and effort, delaying patient care and transport. These failures discourage a repeated fluid triage and assiduous secondary casualty assessments. Vayer et al. also reported that non-advantages are present in scenes with more than 25 casualties.

Vayer et al. suggest in their work that the reliability relies on in the simplicity and on the familiarity with the triage process. They also recommend the addition of more visible geographical information, such as colored flags next to the casualty.

Other research works around triage tag found problems with its design, as the case of Nocera et al. which reports in his work*Australian Disaster Triage: A Colour Maze in the Tower of Babel, 1999* [NG99a]. They reported failures based on a survey applied to emergency departments in Australia. They found that one major problem was the lack of standardization. They distinguished five different models of triage tags among the different emergency departments in the country. This multiplicity of versions might be a problem in MCI scenarios involving different relief units.

Nocera et al. advert that many triage tags were made of perishable materials, leading to mechanical failure under field conditions. In their work, they provide a list of potential problems, mainly related to the design of the cards. Some problems are the impossibility to track and update changes in the casualty's condition because the lack of space. Also, the attachment of the tag is not secure, sometimes dislodging from the patients' neck. They also mention that information might be occulted by blood spots and non-prepared for inclement weather. Nocera et al. also discuss on operational problems. For example, they reported time-consuming problems to document completely the physician triage, they also suggested that the visibility can be easily obstructed. Understanding conflicts with different cards from diverse departments were as well observed. They also suggest that triage tags might interfere with the medical procedures and remark that medical personnel might not use them because they are unfamiliar with the triage tags.

More recent investigations support the mentioned findings, as the one presented by Garner in his work *Documentation and tagging of casualties in multiple casualty incidents*, 2003 [Gar03]. Garner makes an analysis of two MCI scenarios; one occurred in Sioux City, Iowa, involving the crash of a DC-10 aircraft, with 297 persons aboard, and the other Three Rivers Regata. He relates that in the first scenario, health workers decided not to use triage tags in order to save time. The involved health workers in the rescue operation preferred to implement a triage geographical system. It means that the treatment area is sectioned depending on triage categories, and a 210 cm high colored flag identifies each section. Garner also explains that at the Three Rivers Regatta incident, the triage tags were used to record the patient information and diagnose, but not to indicate the triage category. In this way, Garner suggests that the tag may have more application being used as documentation card than being used as tactical reference.

A deeper analysis of the triage tag usability is provided by Käser et al. in their publication *Die Patientenanhängetaschekarte in der medizinischen Gefahrabwehr (The hanging patient bag and card in the emergency medicine), 2012* [KWF12]. They present the results of three emergency drills, involving from thirty to fifty patients, and where they tested the usability of 122 triage tags. The results presented by Käser et al. indicate that 19% of the triage tags were defective. Either the plastic was broken, adding a hazard to the patient and the paramedics or the hole to hold the aglet broke quickly, and many cords were knotted, adding challenges to the paramedics.

They also observed that only 43% of the front side of the tags were used for documentation. Also, only 6% of the tags had information on the rear side, where relevant information could be indicated. In their experiment in 99% of the tags, the coloured triage category was defined, and only in 22%, of them the selected color did not correspond to the last triage class, leading to uncertainty.

Käser et al. suggest, as the above-mentioned research works that unfamiliarity and lack of standard objectives are a reason for failure. They emphasize that to achieve the logistic organization of a rescue operation, the availability of suitable documentation process and effective information flow is indispensable. They state that the abandon of the current triage tag is imminent since there is no other option than to improve it. Data management on a real field requires new and reliable solution that satisfies the necessities of the rescue management.

Despite the mentioned problems, triage tags are still the unique documentation solution. Recent MCI scenarios, as the train accident in Eschede and the mass panic incident at the Love Parade in Duisburg, both in Germany, confirm the impracticality of the tag as a tool to support the tactical planing. Triage tags were partially used to document but not as a reference for the tactical planning. Thus, they only represent a partial solution, but they are too far to be considered a reliable solution to support the continuous demand for information on the ground.

3.1.3 Design Challenges for New MCI Management ICT

The management of MCI scenarios requires new information and communication systems. There is no doubt that the success of the operation organization relies on the information flow and that current tools are only useful in the theory, but not suitable to satisfy the real necessities on the field. Based on the documented experiences and lessons learned accumulated during real MCI, this section describes the conception of new IC solutions for this field.

The information necessity along the organizational and communication chain on the field are the same in principle. Commanders, physicians and paramedics look to dynamically and continuously come up with the answers to: ***who, needs what, from whom, where and who need it first***. Triage tags were conceived to support this consign, but as the experiences show, they are not a suitable solution.

Digital telecommunication represents a real chance to satisfy the demand for data flow during crisis response. Since the beginning of the last century, the development and integration of new and advanced ICT have been a constant. Some of these technological advances are embedded and expert systems, the integration of radio modules with miniaturized sensors and processing units, mobile devices and computers, and networking. Most of the newest technologies have been designed to fulfill daily life conditions, their adaptation to the requirements of the MCI scenarios sets an enormous challenge. Sharoda et al. address this problem in the work *The Usefulness of Information and Communication Technologies in Crisis Response, 2008* [PRAD08]:

> *„Information and communication technologies (ICTs) play a physiological role in coordinating disaster response between pre-hospital services and emergency departments of hospitals. In spite of the advances in these technologies, there remain a variety of challenges to their usage during crisis".*

Shadora et al. deduced from interviews with different emergency departments and emergency medical services, a series of relevant requirements for the design of new ICTs for the management of MCI scenarios. These requirements are discussed as follow:

Structured Data from an unstructured scenario

At MCI scenarios, diverse information at different rate are collected, and this information should be automatically processed, organized and presented in a straightforward manner. In this way commanders, physicians and paramedics can log the required information quickly.

Health workers need mobile and portable devices to introduce and to record data. These devices should be ready for wireless communication. In order to support data transfer and storage, a local area network (LAN) , including access points, gateways and servers, should be available on the incident scenario.

Interoperability and standardization

New technologies should be built following the logistic of the already existing rescue processes; they should also be intuitive and easy to use without a profound previous formation. Documentation should be understandable among health workers from different organizations.

The interoperability between technological platforms from different emergency groups should be ensured, facilitating the information flow and interaction between these groups. An auto-adaptability is required along with the possibility to adjust communication channels. Also, an agreement on the data type and structure is necessary among agencies from different districts and countries.

Abstraction and Push of relevant information

New IT solutions for the MCI scenarios should include features for the auto-processing and abstraction of relevant. In this way, it is possible to filter and present relevant information to the commanders. For example, an automatic data abstraction could inform about the deterioration of the physiological condition of a casualty, an increment on the number of patients with red category, and the arrival of new ambulances.

On the whole and taking the discussed experiences as a basis, state of the art triage tags, paper and manual documentation should be improved. Last advances on ICTs may be, through some adaptation, a reliable solution that satisfies the demand for information during MCI.

Shadora et al. summarized lessons learned and pointed design recommendations for new solutions. They emphasize on the necessity of simple and standard solutions that still allowed the autonomous presentation of well-structured and relevant information of an unstructured scenario.

The communication between the incident commander, authorities and hospitals should be supported. Wireless communication and networking are necessary to support the acquisition, processing, storage and logging of data at the field and from a certain distance. Wireless local area networks (WLAN) and wide area networks (WAN) should be available to support the communication. Moreover, it is not possible to rely on the civilian infrastructure because it can be affected and interrupted by the incident or the incident occurred at non-communicated areas.

Communication during MCI requires an ad hoc solution. Physicians are not ICT experts and do not have the resources to set and to maintain an on-site network. Thus, it should be auto-configurable, robust and energy efficient. In this way, it can be operative along the rescue operation. Different research groups have pursued to build solutions satisfying these requirements. The next section presents and discusses some of them.

Furthermore, new solutions should increase the awareness at the various phases of the organizational chain. At the field, updated medical information to ensure the care provision should be continuously available for paramedics and physician; meanwhile for the commanders, the abstraction of relevant information should be automatically presented.

Embedded electronic technologies make data fusion from sensor-based platforms and human information possible. Different platform have been introduced and studied in a prototype phase by different research. Those systems are discussed in the next section as well.

3.2 Incident Area Networks (IAN)

In the last two decades, an intense research work attempting to bring telecommunication networks to the crisis response field has been done. Logistics and management during MCI scenarios require the organization and interaction of individuals from multiple agencies. Lessons learned as the ones gleaned from 9-11 and Hurricane Katrina, shows that the lack of interoperability between different agencies has been a problem to achieve a common plan [KN07] [MB07] [RPA+09]. Thus, standard and flexible ground intercommunication and long distance communication between incidents commander, authorities and hospital are necessary.

Moreover, MCI requires ad-hoc network solutions, independent of civilian communication infrastructure [GMS+07a]. These solutions must be easily deployable, autonomous and auto-configurable [CSK10] [KRS+09]. Since the middle of 1990, different research institutions have conceived and explored, solutions fulfilling these requirements, naming them *incident area networks (IAN)* [MJT00, Del09].

Figure 3.2 shows a general concept of IAN and how they could link and cover information demand between different agents at different levels of the organizational chain. Different research groups have already pursuit to solve different challenges of IAN at different communications levels; the next sections discuss the most representative.

3.2.1 Telecommunications Infrastructure

As mentioned above, the implementation of customized information and communications solutions is the first mandate to solve the communication problems during MCI scenarios. More portable radio modules, accessible costs and energy efficient, make the conception of suitable IAN possible [LMFj+04]. As depicted in figure 3.2 the coexistence of hybrid

LAN and WAN technologies is required to satisfy the information demand on all organization phases.

Researchers have approached the scenario bringing different communication technologies and network topologies. Some of them have involved hybrid terrestrial and satellite communication and others, the newest protocols for autonomous wireless sensor networks (AWSN) .

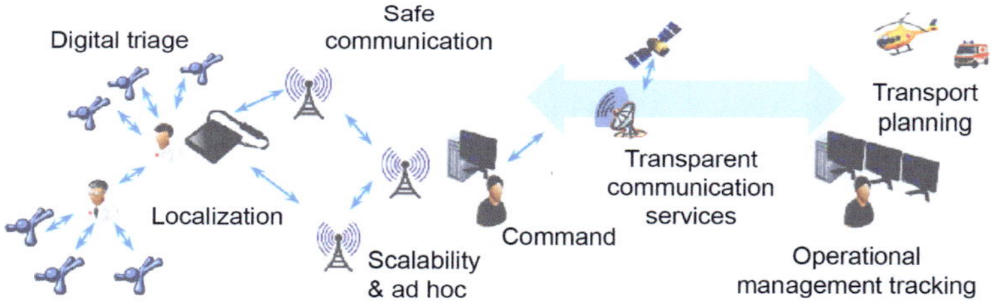

Figure 3.2: Incident area network SeCoServ2

Hybrid Terrestrial and Satellite Communication Networks

In 1976, the National Aeronautics and Space Administration (NASA) performed one of the first attempts to study the feasibility to support communications on MCI scenarios with satellite technology. During the simulation, of an airport emergency incident, satellite communication was used to allow the assessment of a burn patient. Portable based telecommunication systems included video cameras, two-way voice communication and the Application Technology Satellite-6 (ATS-6) and Hermes satellite (communication technology satellite CTS). The study evidenced the value for satellite technologies to assist significant urgencies, supporting medical organization and the assessment and triaging of mass casualties [CES82].

The advantages of satellite communication were evidenced later during real MCI situations. In 1979, after a tornado in Wichita Falls, Texas, caused 1000 casualties and different damages including local communication services over an area of 16 km^2. Only after the next day, a single emergency telephone connection was established via ATS-6 and a jeep-mounted satellite transceiver. This experimental equipment allowed to connect Wichita with the Texas authorities successfully in Austin and the first response local governmental agencies.

Another story of success occurred during the earthquake at Mexico City in 1985. The ATS-3 from NASA was physiological to provide voice communication supporting the relief activities of the American Red Cross and the Pan American Health Organization. The ATS-3 was crucial to support the field communications since the earthquake disrupted all local communications. Within 24 hours, ATS-3 prioritize the communication traffic involving disaster management and rescue operations.

Other satellite technologies that provided communication support during MCI scenarios through the 1990 decade were: INMARSAT, COMSAT , Orion, GTE Spacenet, G-Star and ACTS . They supported image, video and audio transmission, as well as specialized applications for computer tomography and ultrasound. Some of them started to integrate IP communication to support internet communication, web-browsing and e-mail transfer. Also, specialized network management was incorporated as ATM and ISDN.

Today two satellite networks are available: geostationary (GEO) and low Earth orbit (LEO). Geostationary satellites are in fixed positions 36,000 km above the Earth. They provide a globe region with a variety of communication services, including audio, video and broadband data. They link with ground bases with vast antennas or mobile terminals [GB99].

In contrast, LEO satellites are not static and are they move in a range of 780 km and 1,500 km above the Earth. Since they are much closer to the Earth than GEO satellites, ground transmitter and receiver power requirements, size and costs are reduced. LEO satellites are significant for disaster management since they can operate from any part of the world at any time, without depending on communications base stations. However, they only support basic communication, as an audio and low-speed data transmission rates.

Despite the fact that peer-to-peer analog voice communication is still popular on the ground, some MCI situations might need larger coverage. Specialized terrestrial networks to support long range coverage for voice and low-speed data transfer have evolved. It is the case of TETRA (terrestrial trunked radio), conceived primarily to support communication among government agencies and emergency services during MCI scenarios. The introduction of TETRA represents an option over satellite communication. Because it is in lower frequency bands, it allows extended geographic coverage, significantly above than ordinary walkie-talkies [BCW07a].

Another important system is GSM (global system for mobile communications), which has been developed since 1980 parallel to satellite and specialized terrestrial communications. It has been conceived to satisfy consumer mobile communication necessities. Today, GSM permits with its bandwidth high data transfer rate. It might support by antenna stations or fiber optic networks within urbanizations. GSM networks are vulnerable to disasters. However, telephone services might recover with the support of satellite links [FWC+08].

In addition, portable technologies, as the BGAN (Broadband Global Area Network) terminals, support satellite internet network or telephony where civilian telephone infrastructure is missing. The terminals link to the GEO INMARSAT satellite constellation, and it requires a line-of-sight to the satellite. The main purpose of BGAN terminals is to support background IP for internet and telephone voice. Similar to BGAN the DVB-RCS terminals support digital video broadcasting via satellite [spa].

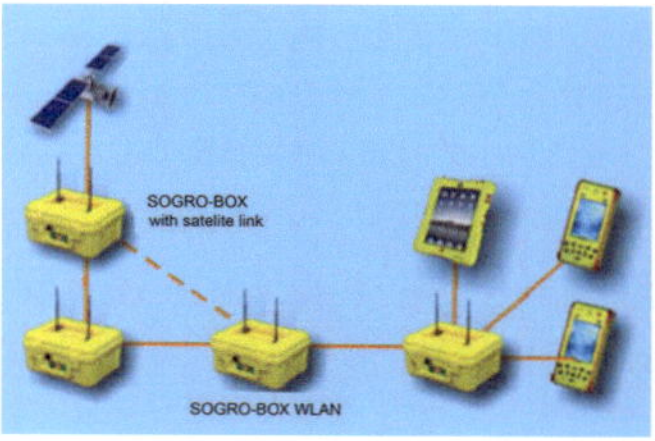

(a) SOGRO IAN wireless communication cells

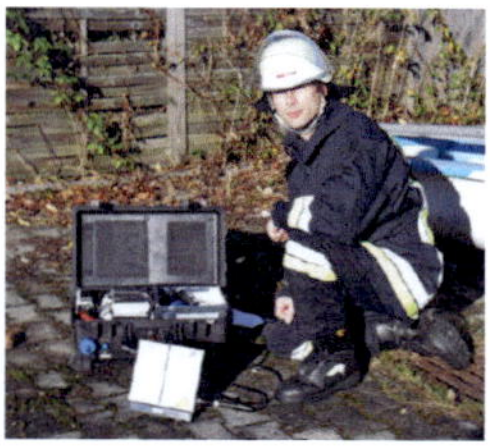

(b) e-Triage wireless communication cell

Figure 3.3: IAN wireless communication cells of projects SOGRO and e-Triage [EL12, AKGM+11]

Research projects have attempted to join all these technologies in order to satisfy image, video, audio, text, web-browsing, and e-mail communication within the incident area during MCI. Examples of these projects are WISECOM [BCW07a, BCW07b, BCC+11] and WIISARD [CGP+12, LCG+06, BCK+07] from United States and SOGRO [EL12, EFK13] and e-Triage [AKGM+11, DEA+11, GMD10] from Germany. The main idea is to deploy communication cells on the field to support ground and remote communications. The cells have been extended with WLAN capabilities to support the transfer of digital data on the ground. Figure 3.3 depicts the communication cells from SOGRO and e-Triage. These communication cells, when interacting with mobile computing devices, support the digital documentation and automatic report between the EP on the ground and the commander center. In this way, it is possible to leave aside paper documentation, apparently adding an advantage to the information management task.

Autonomous Wireless Sensor Networks

Autonomous wireless sensor network (AWSN) are commonly conformed by devices, popularly known as motes. Small-size, low-power consumption and radio communication capabilities distinguish them. Miniaturization of communication modules, sensors technologies, control processor units, power units, among others, combined with integrated platforms, has contributed to the development of WSN. Their reduced size and low-power consumption characteristics make feasible the production of wearable embedded devices and the interaction with portable computers [LMFj+04].

During the last two decades, different wireless technologies and standard protocols for wireless communication in LAN have evolved. Mobile and portable computers, sensors, along with wireless communication standards such as IEEE 802.11 and IEEE 802.15, have made possible the high rate wireless transmission of any digitalized data. Wireless communication technologies are present in countless areas of daily life, and they may represent a revolutionary progress in the management of MCI scenarios.

IEEE 802.11 standard is the compendium of specifications for media access control and the physical layer. It defines the implementation of WLAN-devices in the frequency bands of 2.4, 3.6, 5 and 60 GHz, commonly known as Wi-Fi. Palmtop computer, ordinarily known as personal digital assistant, combines the computational and radio function into a portable device. They support Wi-Fi connections and allow the transmission of digital information [WLA12]. The introduction of mobile handheld devices into the emergency field can significantly reduce the documentation effort and the voice communication traffic.

In contrast, the IEEE 802.15 standard establishes a series of specifications for wireless LAN with shorter coverage range. They are known as wireless personal area network (WPAN) [WPA05]. IEEE 802.15 encapsulates different groups of technologies, for example, 802.15. define the Bluetooth protocol and 802.15.4 the Zigbee. Zigbee is conceived mainly for low-power consumption transmission. Zigbee allows long time operation rates, even for years [ZIG14]. Specification for body area networks (BAN) are also included and registered as the standard IEEE 802.15.6. It sets the requirements for the communication between devices and sensors in, or around the body.

Standard communication protocols support interoperability from the physical to the network layer between different devices regardless the manufacturer. The challenge for the interoperability relies on now from the transport to the application layer of the open system intercommunication (OSI) model.

During the last ten years, different research groups studied the potential of WSN and their possible introduction to the management of MCI situations.They have approached the on-site communication problem with the implementation of different AWSN solutions, integrating various of the above-mentioned protocols. Most of them have provided the physicians and the paramedics with handheld computers and built on-site a WLAN, supporting in this way the automatic documentation of relevant information. Other projects have gone further and have substituted the triage tags with an electronic version, extended with physiological and physiological sensors. The addition of medical sensor allows a continuous monitoring of the physiological status of the casualty. Table 3.1 lists the research projects and their corresponding platforms and technologies.

The challenge to develop AWSN suitable for the hostility of MCI scenarios relies on producing ad hoc solutions satisfying some of the requirements presented in section 3.1.3. Mainly, they have to be simple, intuitive, comfortable and practical to use; since there is no time available to configure or to build the network on-site. Moreover, health workers are not prepared to solve technical problems. Thus, the network must be independent and auto-configurable [CSK10, RHKW11] . Autonomous network management should automatically establish links between end-nodes, access points and servers. In this way, information from end-nodes can reach the servers or end-points dynamically, independently of its high mobility among the incident area. WSN for MCI scenarios must have a decentralized topology, and a unit server or single end-point approaches do not represent a reliable solution. Decentralized or mesh networks are a robust approach, which avoids failure of single end-point communication technologies [MGW+06]. Another point to consider is that communication bandwidth for IEEE 802.15 standards is highly limited on low-power radio modules. Prioritization among the message type is necessary, e.g., information coming from a severe injured patient must have priority over a non-injured casualty.

Table 3.1: Recent research projects and WSN technologies for MCI scenarios

System	Network	Patient-tracking device	Other Device	Reference
AID-N	Zigbee, WiFi, GSM, Satellite	Pulse oximeter, blood pressure, ECG	Hand-held computer	[GMS+07b]
WIISARD	WIFI mesh network, GSM, Satellite	Pulse oximeter	Hand-held computer	[CGP+12]
WISECOM	WiFi, UMTS, WiMAX, TETRA, GSM	-	Hand-held computer	[BKS96]
CODEBlue	Zigbee, WiFi	Pulse oximeter, heart rate, ECG	PDA	[MFJWM04]
SOGRO	WiFi, UMTS, TETRA, BGAN	RFID armbands	PDA	[EFK13]
E-Triage	WLAN, GSM/GPRS, TETRA	RFID triage card	Hand-held computer	[AKGM+11]
ALARM	UMTS, GPRS, Satellite	RFID triage card	PDA	[LDWS12]
ARTEMIS	WIFI	Hand-held with ECG and Pulse oximeter	-	[MGW+03]
eTriage	Zigbee, WiFi	SpO2, HR, Breath rate	Hand-held computer	[HUY11]

Because the large number of casualties in disaster situations, network scalability may also be an issue. Network management should be possible over extended areas and for a large number of sensors. Low-power consumption is also to consider, nodes must operate along the whole rescue operation.

In brief, self-organization is a crucial attribute for WSN especially for MCI scenarios. Four aspects describe a self-organizing WSN: *self-configuration*, *self-healing*, *self-optimization* and *self-protection*. During MCI scenarios, the WSN must provide reliable data transfer over a noisy, error-prone and variable channels. WSN is not failure-free, so fault tolerance and self-healing are, therefore, to be considered for their implementation at MCI scenarios, along with energy management [CSK10]. Self-optimization to establish the less power-consuming communication also plays an important role in the development of WSN.

Zigbee (IEEE 802.15.4) has self-organization properties. Thus, it has been commonly selected among different research groups. Zigbee has been developed by the Zigbee Alliance for low-power and short range applications. It is characterized by the versatility to support automatically different network topologies, included mesh. It is also considered suitable for the MCI events due to its capability to handle networks up to 1000 nodes [ZIG14].

3.2.2 Real-time Information Aggregation & Visualization

As discussed in the last section, wireless communications and sensor networks are capable of revolutionizing the data collection process at large emergency situations. Wireless technologies allow the automatic and real-time data transfer. Mobile computers can then be used to introduce patient information or triage information, in the same way as in the triage tags. The commander can receive the information automatically and visualize it at the command center.

In research projects, paramedics and physicians have been provided with hand-held devices to support data collection, patient identification and to access already documented information about the patient. In the same way, specific software applications have been developed to analyze and organize incident information and to present it to the commanders.

Handheld Computer for Physicians & Paramedics

PDAs have become popular in the last 15 years, providing a new form to introduce, organize, store, access and transfer data. These portable computers allow people to connect wirelessly to data servers and internet. Special software applications for different purposes have been developed for different operating systems for PDA , e.g. word processor, agenda, e-mail, web-browser, teleconference, camera, etc. [DAGM12].

In the case of emergency medicine, digital protocols have been implemented for PDAs. When a typical emergency occurs, paramedics can digitally document relevant information about the casualty. PDAs are commonly used during individual emergency services, there paramedics can introduce the diagnosis of the casualty and generate a digital record. However, they are not used for MCI cases, due to the lack of connectivity in a scenario far from communication infrastructure [GAR+05].

On the other hand, PDAs have been used in all research projects related to the implementation of IAN. Physicians can introduce in specific SW for disaster management, information about the patient and the triage information, more applications and advantages are explained in [KCB+06, NK07, MFJWM04, MGW+06, GMS+07b]. The SW has been typically built based on the triage tags protocols so that the process is still familiar to the physicians.

In order to identify the patients, PDAs are extended with bar code or radio frequency identification (RFID) readers, meaning that patients should be tagged with bar code or RFID tags. Figure 3.4 depicts various examples of PDAs implemented by the different research groups.

Data Visualization at Commander Center

Digital patient data collection constitutes a step forward towards data handling at the commander center. Senior emergency physician, organizational and incident commanders, can log and visualize data coming from the field automatically. They do not need anymore to organize information on whiteboards; now specialized software applications can provide information about who needs what, from whom, where and who need it first [KRS+09, RHKW11].

Different research groups have developed different SW applications by attending the necessities of the MCI management. They present the statistics about the incident, including the number of victims and the number of victims by category. Also, screens display specific information about each. Every time that a patient triage occurs, they receive the information on their devices, in this manner the voice communication traffic is reduced, and the paper protocols are annulated [MJT00, MW12, DGL07].

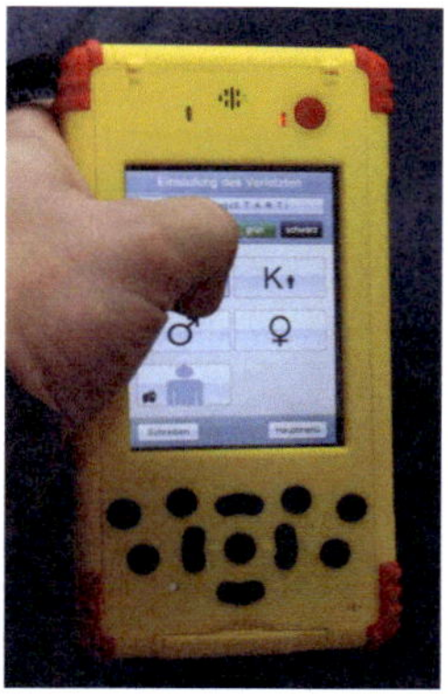

(a) PDA SOGRO

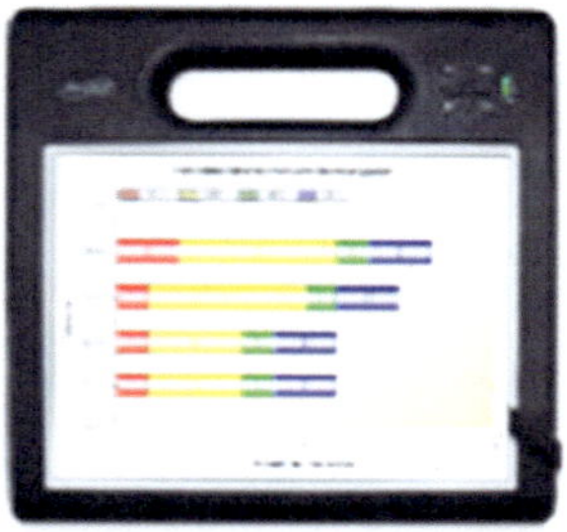

(b) Tablet e-Triage

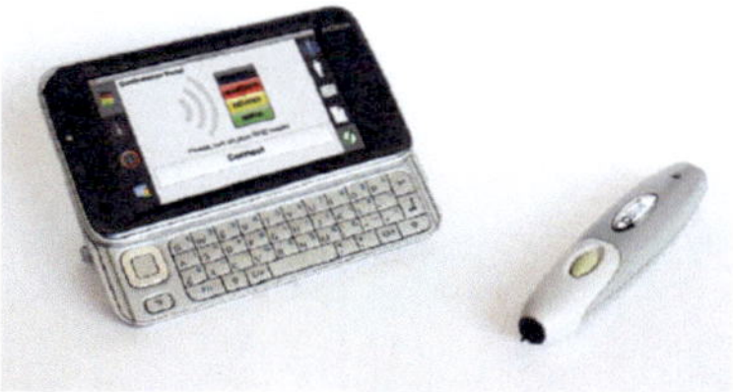

(c) eTraige

Figure 3.4: PDA and tablets for digital docummentation during MCI [EL12, DEA+11]

In the case where electronic devices with physiological sensors substitute triage tags, commanders can also follow the ECG signals, HR and SpO2 information among other in real-time. Some electronic triage tags or PDAs are extended with localization modules, allowing the incident managers to locate casualties on the field [CMV12].

Real-time data visualization of medical and tactical information improves the logistical plan, accelerating the decision-making process based on more accurate and precise information [FMB07, GSMF05] . Software applications for the commander are interactive and allow them to organize information, including the transport logistic or the distribution of medical care on the incident site. Examples of tools for the operation command, implemented by different research projects, are depicted in figure 3.5.

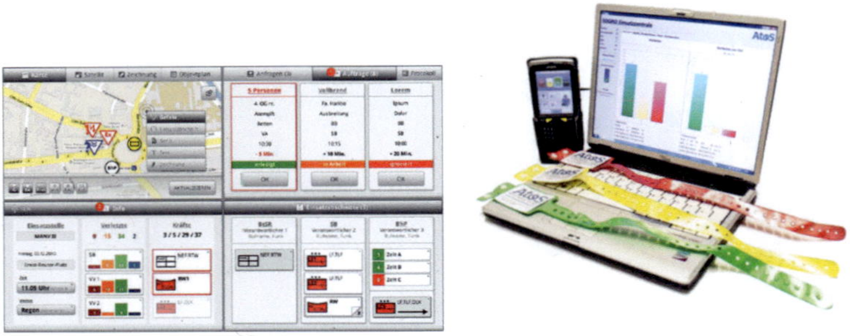

(a) eTriage (b) SOGRO

Figure 3.5: Real-time visualization platform for MCI scenarios

3.2.3 Electronic Triage Tags

Aside the documentation and communication process, paper triage tags have been also extended with electronic and digital information modules. In some cases, the triage tag have been provided with passive RFID tags to support the digital identification of patients. Triage tags have been kept as a backup in case the electronic support fails. In other cases, the triage tag have been completely substituted by an electronic card. The tag is an electronic mote in an AWSN, and it can transmit different information depending on the integrated modules, as physiological patient information or its localizations.

Non-active Triage Tag

Some commercial triage tags include bar codes for rapid patient identification, but this can be easily damaged or occulted by spots, like blood. RFID is an alternative to identifying patients and to relate the patients with the correct information at data servers [FL, ISOF06, JRG+12, NAC+11].

Since the middle of 1990s, radio frequency identification have been com-mercialized. It is based on the mutual induction discovered by Faraday, which is the basis for powering passive tag by near electromag-netic fields. RFID requires two elements, an active reader and a passive backscatter tag. The passive tag has an antenna and integrated chip circuitry. The antenna performs two primary functions; it harvests energy from the reader signal and communicates back the id to the reader. The integrated chip is a basic oscillator circuit that generates a wave depending on the stored id. The user device produces the wave to energize the passive tag and acquires and interprets the signal coming back from the RFID tag [AI08]. Figure 3.11(a) exemplifies how the RFID works and show some example of tags.

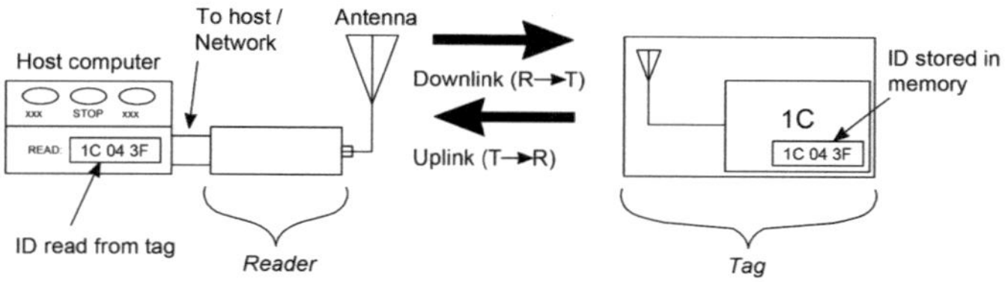

(a) RFID concept

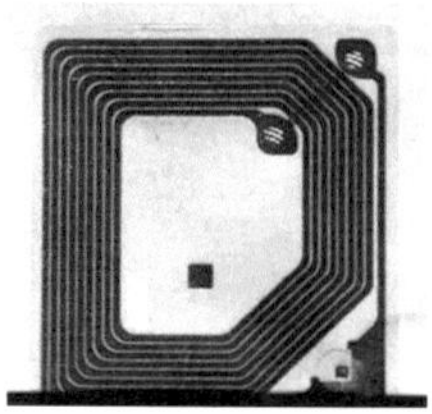

(b) RFID tag

Figure 3.6: RFID system and tag [AI08]

Research projects working with non-active tag replaced the actual tags by colored wristbands with RFID tags or extended them only attaching an RFID tag [LDWS12, AEMK12, EL12]. PDAs have RFID readers to support a rapid and digital identification and tracking of the casualties.

Figure 3.7 presents the triage tag with RFID capabilities explored by the projects SOGRO and e-Triage.

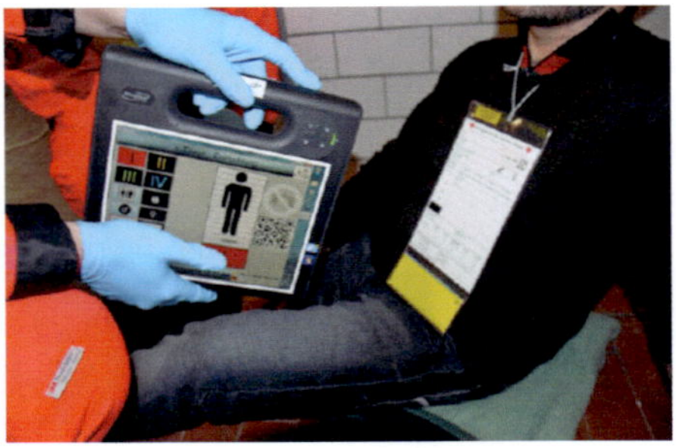

Figure 3.7: Triage tag with RFID from e-Triage project [DEA+11]

Active Triage Tag

In section 3.2.1 some research projects introducing WSN infrastructure to the incident area were mentioned. Some of that projects have opted to substitute the ordinary paper triage tag by electronic motes. These motes are portable embedded platforms, which integrate different modules, as physiological parameters control and localization. An advantage of active triage tags is that they facilitate the collection of casualty information, they frequently update relevant data about the patient, and they facilitate its positioning. A constant monitoring is appropriate for MCI scenarios. It avoids the dependency on the available physicians to get patient data. Also the consistency of the reports improves through a continuous and automatic data update [MCMYC11, KNO11, SHS+11].

Active Vital Parameters Monitoring

Active-monitoring of physiological parameters, e.g. ECG, SpO2, HR have been integrated with active triage tags. In Table 3.1 research projects with electronic triage tag and the corresponding technologies for physiological monitoring are listed.

Active localization

Two approaches technological approaches for the dynamic localization of patients are now presented. One includes GPS and the other uses reference nodes on the ground. These nodes broadcast their fixed position to the mobile motes. Based on the fixed position and the received signal strength indication (RSSI) from at least three references it is possible to estimate through triangulation the position of the mobile mote.

- *Global Position System (GPS)*is a space-based satellite positioning and navigation system. The U.S. Department of Defense implemented the GPS program at the beginning of 1970's. Only until its completion in 1993, the twenty-four satellites constellation covered all the globe. This system can provide continuous position and timing information to ground portable devices.
  GPS functionality depends on three elements: the satellites, the ground-based control stations and the user devices. Satellites are in six orbital planes, between 20,200 km and 26,560 km above the Earth. Four satellites are in each orbit, assuring that from four to ten satellites are visible at any place worldwide. Additionally, only four satellites are necessary to calculate the localization of GPS receiver device [ER02].
  The ground control stations are around the world and are advocated to track the satellites integrity and to maintain their operability. The user devices have antennas and IC modules to process signals coming from the satellite. Two carrier frequencies, two digital protocols and the navigation message compose the GPS Signal, which contains the position, velocity, altitude, and error information.
  The carrier frequencies and the digital protocols are used to determine the distance between the satellite and the receiver. The distance to three satellites is required at least in order to estimate the position based on the resection concept. But four reference satellites are necessary to locate the receiver in the intersection of four spheres, determined by the distance between the receiver and the satellite. Figure 3.8 presents GPS IC receivers.

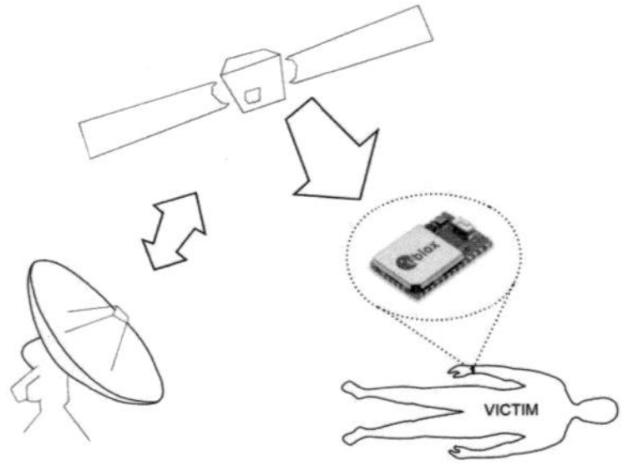

Figure 3.8: GPS receiver and patient localization (http://www.tomtom.com, http://www.ublox.com)

- *RSSI Triangulation*, similar to the GPS intersection concept, the RSSI from fixed nodes is used to determine the position of a mobile node. RSSI is an indication of the signal strength commonly expressed in [dBm]. It is dependent on the distance between neighbored and the physical channel properties among them [CS09].

  There are many approaches to process and calculate the distances. One is given by Chandra-Sekaran et al. in the work *Efficient Resource Estimation During Mass Casualty Emergency Response Based on a Location Aware Disaster Aid Network* [CSFK+08]. They suggest that the mobile node broadcast a beacon and that the neighbored anchor nodes reply with their position and the average of RSSI. The mobile node requires the position of at least three neighbored reference nodes to determine its position. The estimated distance results from an imaginary radius, and the area resulting from the intersection will indicate the area where the node is located [Kun].

  Another similar approach is presented by Shnayder et al. in *Sensor Networks for Medical Care* [SCL+05]. They offer an empirical solution based on a look-up table with a predefined position of fixed nodes. The mobile node receives from the reference nodes repeatedly a beacon message containing the averages RSSI. Then it references its position to the fixed node and determines its position into a 3D space.

  RSSI triangulation has the advantage that it is suitable for indoor and outdoor scenarios, whereas GPS is suitable only for outdoor.

However, RSSI triangulation requires setting anchor nodes among the incident area, and it may not be practicable since the localization accuracy increases with the number of reference nodes.

3.3 Remote Monitoring of Casualty's Vital Signs

Active triage tags enable the remote and continuous monitoring of patients. Many developed triage tags might have physiological sensors, making possible to assess the physiological and physiological condition of the casualty. In this way, emergency doctors can track patient's progress remotely, or they can get alarms based on the sensor information. More-over, some active triage tags also determine the triage category automat-ically. Active triage tags keep the commanders informed supporting the decision- making on the field continuously, without depending on the number of physicians performing the triage and assessment on the field.

This section presented various examples of active triage tags and how they take advantage of the physiological sensors in different ways. Some of them present only raw values, without analyzing them for the abstraction of relevant events. While other might perform some analysis and evaluation to recognize critical conditions and generate some alarms; the other can determine the triage status automatically. Automatic evaluation of physiological state occurs similar to know triage algorithms, as START. Next sections depict different approaches that evaluates auto-matically and reports dynamically on the physiological condition of the victims.

3.3.1 Automatic Report and Evaluation of Vital Condition

The projects CODEBlue [Ina11b], AID-N [GGW+06] and WIISARD [BGD + 06] developed active triage tags. They were able to transmit physiological parameters, some were able also to recognize certain critical status and alarm the physicians automatically.

CODEBlue project developed an active triage tag integrating an OEM pulse oximeter and electrocardiogram. Physicians and commanders can log to the patient's information and track live the SpO2, HR and ECG signal. There is no evidence that the members of CODEBlue designed algorithms to evaluate the patient condition automatically. During MCI, despite the advantage of logging physiological parameters and signals remotely, the effort of the decision-makers augmented since they had to analyze the data of each patient [MFJWM04].

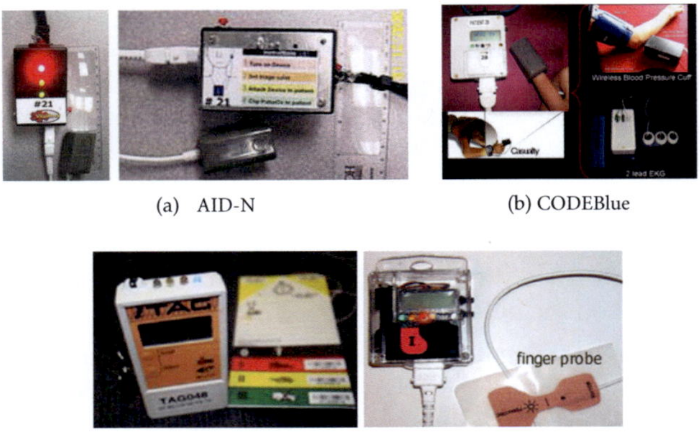

(a) AID-N (b) CODEBlue

(c) WISSARD Tag (d) WISSARD Tag

Figure 3.9: Active triage tags with physiological sensors [MGB+06]

The WISSARD project introduces two active triage tags, one with physiological sensors; this tag is only for clinical injured patients. Physicians determine which patients require continuous monitoring of their physiological signs. They can log the information of the tag to observe the SpO2 and HR. In this case, as occurs with the approach of CODEBlue, the application only shows the raw values and commanders must go through lists or tables to process and evaluate the status of each patient. This task clearly adds an extra effort to the data management a the commander center [CBP+09].

In the case of project AID-N, a post-processing and evaluation of the physiological parameters is performed. In this way, particular clinical situations are filtered and recognized. AID-N developed an active triage tag similar to CODEBlue's tag but also including non-invasive blood pressure. In Table 3.2 the conditions to set the alarm are depicted [GGW+06].

Table 3.2: AID-N alert detection parameters

Alert Type	Detection Parameter
low SpO2	SpO2 <90%
bradycardia	HR <40 bpm
tachycardia	HR >150 bpm
HR change	$\|\Delta HR/5min\| > 19\%$
HR stability	max HR variability from 4 past readings <10%
HR change	systolic or diastolic change >±11%

The PDA of the physicians informs about these relevant events automatically. The thresholds are semi-automatically configurable either based on information introduced by a physician, as age and gender; or on sensor information as pressure and temperature. Physicians can log the physiological signals in order to perform a deeper analysis of the patient condition.

3.3.2 Automatic Triage

The manual analysis of physiological parameters or the interpretation of warnings might be tedious on the field. Two projects have gone beyond and provided a sensor-based triage. The project ARTEMIS from U.S. [MGW+03] and eTriage from Japan [HUY11] perform an automatic evaluation of the physiological parameters SpO2 and HR and determine the triage category automatically. The automatic evaluation is based on the START algorithm, explained in section 2.1.2. The automatic abstraction of the patient condition based on a familiar process might be a more reliable solution compared to the approaches presented in the last section.

The project ARTEMIS provides a solution for military casualties where the objective is to provide a remote triage reference so that the doctors must not go on the field and put their self under risk [WMB03]. The triage tag consists on a PDA with a pulse oximeter. When the device recognizes a non-normal physiological state, soldiers must provide information on the PDA's screen, indicating its walking capacity, in this way it also evaluates the consciousness. If a soldier does not answer, physiological parameters are tested to provide a triage category [CM06, WMBA04].

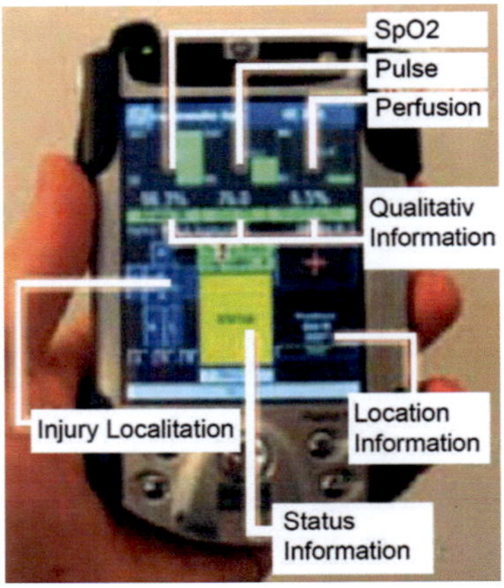

Figure 3.10: ARTEMIS PDA for self triage and automatic triage

They define the triage categories as fuzzy classes: adequate and low. Table 3.3 explains the conditions to evaluate the parameters and establish the triage category [MGW^+03, CBP^+09].

Table 3.3: ARTEMIS - automatic triage conditions [WMB03]

Triage category	Parameter condition			
	walk	**concious**	**SpO2**	**HR**
green / minimal	yes	yes	>70%	>40 bpm
yellow / delayed	no	yes	>70 %	>40 bpm
red / urgent	no	-	<70%	<40 bpm
black / expectant	no	no	abscent	-

The Japanese project eTriage also evaluates various physiological parameters to classify the severity of the casualty according to the START algorithm. Similar to the project WIISARD, in eTriage two different cards, are proposed. They define one tag as the full-triage tag, conceived for the monitoring of severely injured patients, and the light-triage tag with the purpose to track the less injured casualties. The full-triage version estimates the SpO2, HR and the breath rate. It integrates a pulse oximeter, and to measure the air flow and air rate a cannula must be placed inside the nose. The light version only tracks the SpO2 and HR. Table 3.4 depicts the different conditions to determine the triage category. If the tag has defined a new triage category, it will emit a visual and audible alarm, and then the physician has to confirm or correct the new category [MSYI11, SHS+11, SHS+13].

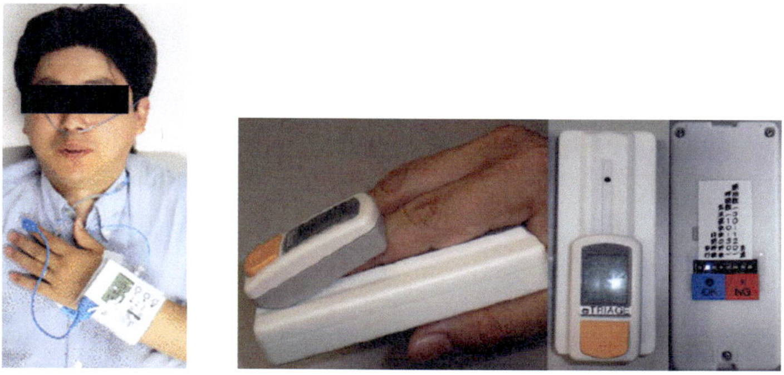

(a) eTriagae full version

(b) eTriage light version

Figure 3.11: Japanese eTriage automatic triage devices [MIS+12]

Table 3.4: eTriage - Automatic Triage Condition [SHS+13]

Parameter	Triage	Condition
Pulse rate [bpm]	Category I red	<50 or >120
	Category II yellow	50-60 or 100-120
	Category III green	60-100
SpO2 [%]	Category I red	<90
	Category II yellow	90 - 96
	Category III green	96 - 100

There is no evidence on how practical is to have two different type of tags on the field since it might require a change of device if the condition of the patients varies from non-critical to critical. The eTriage project does not provide documentation on how it is affecting the task of the physicians when they have to affirm continually that the triage tag have established a new class correctly. Neither ARTEMIS nor eTriage provide a real characterization of the accuracy of their algorithms.

3.4 Summary

Paper triage cards, voice communication and paper protocols and whiteboards are not suitable to support the demand for information during MCIs. In the last years, many research projects had attempted to introduce ICT to these scenarios, supporting the information exchange between the different actors on the field. New ICTs are welcome by rescue personnel. However, there is still room for the optimization. Next chapter presents a novel solution to continue support incident officers with their management activities. The new concept is the result of the analysis of the state of the art and different discussions with experts in the field.

4 Conception of Novel Wearable Platform for Remote Monitoring of Casualties

The last chapter overviews the state of the art and new technological approaches, both to support the first response at MCI scenarios. The focus of these technologies is to attend the demand for information and to assist the communication on the field. Paper triage cards, paper documentation and voice communication are the conventional techniques, but they are not sufficient. Thus, new research projects on this matter have presented a series of solutions based on the latest advances on ICT. They cover different phases of the communication such as communication on the field, communication between paramedics, physicians, commander; and communication between the incidents and external actors such as hospitals and authorities.

New wireless networks, portable computers and miniaturized physiological sensors, represent a more reliable solution to support the communication problems of health workers at the incident area. The objective is to achieve a more accurate operational plan of the rescue and paramedic forces. Various research projects in this field have demonstrated how these technologies are welcome by rescue units, proving that they can be slowly introduced as daily tools for the command of rescue operations.

The different approaches presented in the last chapter introduce the potential of the integrated technologies, however, they do not take full advantage of them. Additionally, in the case of projects with electronic triage tags and an active evaluation of physiological parameters, do not offer a clear explanation of the acceptance or reliability of their developed algorithms. They only present them as an advantageous concept, but do not provide information about their classification or triage accuracy. They do not provide information about the impact of new alerts on the field.

This chapter discusses a new possibility to implicate new ICT technologies in the management of MCI scenarios appropriately. As well, this chapter discusses the conception of a new solution, following a user-centered design strategy. In this way, the experience of experts in the management of MCI scenarios is the basis of the specification of the new solution. In addition, this chapter presents the collection and analysis of requirements for the specification of the new platform. Finally, the idea of a new wearable platform to support the tactical and medical management on the MCI field is presented.

4.1 Tactical Data Abstraction for MCI Management

The implementation of mobile computers and wireless LAN infrastructure at the incident area aims to support the acquisition and documentation of casualty's information. Information about the casualties is better organized and presented automatically to commanders and physicians. However, the information collection rate still depends on the personnel responsible for generating it. In fact, only the emergency physicians can report the triage category and the diagnosis. Therefore, the information flow is only triggered when the doctor on the field inputs it, and consequently the collection process is discontinuous. If the number of casualties is much larger than the number of paramedics, the information demand will not be satisfied even the new technologies.

In the case of implementing active triage tags, the intermittent information flow problem can be handled. The active triage tag with physiological sensors or localization modules can monitor the casualty continuously and inform about it. A constant flow of information must be tactically managed. The amounts of information can lead to overwhelmed health workers, being contradictory to the main objective, which is to present the right information at the right moment. Experts state that only through a dynamic, intuitive and modular information system it is possible to find who needs what, from whom, where and who need it first. The usability of new information technologies is only performant when the presented information is relevant and simple to understand.

4.1.1 Specifications for new MCI Management ICT

Last chapter provided an overview of the application and usability of different new ICT technologies for disaster management. The conclusion of the last decade efforts is that the implementation of wireless infrastructure and digital communication presents an advantage, its potential to assist the management of resources on the field is also clear.

However, the mentioned research projects only provided evidence of the technical feasibility to implement these technologies. They study their impact on the operation's logistics neither the usability of information. For example, there is not enough evidence to prove that passive triage tags are enough to cover the information demand on the field. There is also no evidence to demonstrate that active triage tags are giving accurate information, or whether the form they present the information is useful for the paramedics. Diverse information is necessary at different phases of the MCI coordination, and the logistics behind the information management have not yet properly attended.

The generation of new IC technologies for the mass casualty scenario requires paying more attention to the end user experiences. Until now, MCI scenarios have been mainly seen as an experimental field based on where to test the feasibility and robustness of communication infrastructure. In order to provide a real solution, an integral strategy, where stakeholders participate as the center of the design, must be put into practice. A new solution should provide a reliable mechanism for data abstraction. Information is only usable if it is reliable and significant. Thus, the information process should be familiar and transparent to the end user.

The main challenges to providing a new and more suitable platform are the abstraction of relevant and accurate information, and to achieve a simple and familiar information process.

Abstraction of Relevant and Accurate Information

The use of paper documentation and voice communication limits the communication process at the incident area. Projects as e-Triage and SOGRO implement inactive triage tags supported by RFID. Despite they provided automatic and organized digitalized documentation through PDA's, they only support and reflect the actual communication process; where they depend on the availability of personnel on the field to collect information. The information flow from the field might have the same rate as the actual communication process. Figure 4.1 depicts and compare these information systems and communication methods, the intermittent information flow can be observed.

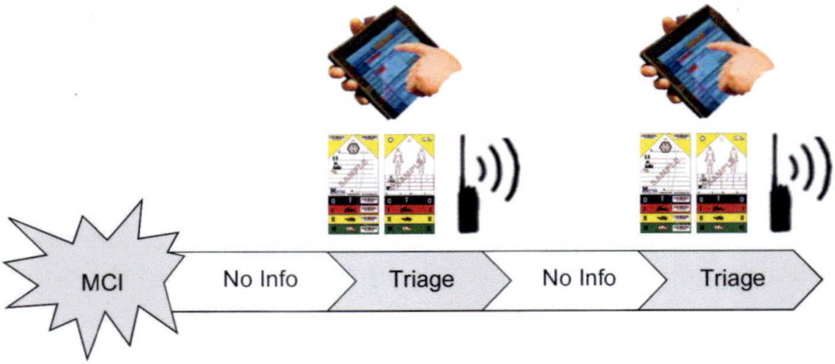

Figure 4.1: Intermmitent information flow at MCI scenarios

In chapter 2.2.1 it is learned that the physiology of the trauma patient tends to fast deterioration if they do not receive prompt attention. In the case of these technologies, the characterization of the patients is dependent on the availability of physicians at the incident area. The accuracy of the casualty's information is also a time-dependent parameter, if it is not constantly updated or revised, it loses creditability and would not be usable.

In contrast, projects as WIISARD, AID-N and eTriage (Japan) included active triage to make the constant monitoring of the patient possible. They present physiological information in tables, but while an MCI scenario, the list of patients can be very long, and physicians do not have the time to review all raw values for each patient. Active triage tags constantly inform about the patient condition and its localization, but the form and amount of information could overwhelm the physicians and commanders. These projects have created algorithms to filter the information and set alarms, but alarms can also overwhelm the physicians if they are not accurate and relevant, see figure 4.2.

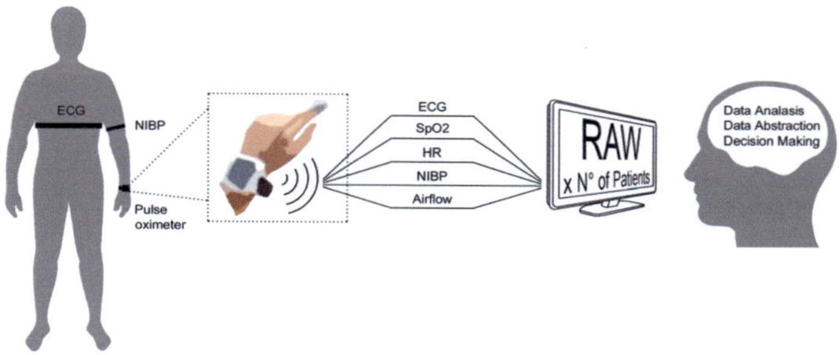

Figure 4.2: Physiological raw data might overwhelm incident officers

In the case of the automatic triage performed by the active tag from eTriage, an audible alarm suggests the nearby physicians that the triage category might have changed. The physician has to verify the alarm and confirm or correct the status. This new verification process will be unfamiliar to the normal process besides adding tasks at the incident area, representing clearly a disadvantage.

Moreover, these projects do not offer information about the accuracy and the variance of the occurrence of the alerts. Thus, it is possible to imagine and depict a scenario where the doctors are overwhelmed by the new alert system. The objective of implementing these new technologies must go further than only the demonstration of its ability to accelerate the information and documentation process as it happens in the projects discussed in chapter 3. It also has to analyze the impact on the ordinary logistic process. The user acceptance should be questioned, unfamiliarity, as explained in section 3.1.3 is a right to reject a new platform. Particularly the introduction of new tasks, which ends overwhelming the physicians would be a reason to refute the introduction of new solutions.

Simple and Standard Information Process

In order to take full advantage of new portable computing, embedded systems, wireless infrastructure and digital information, requires the conception of a tactic strategy to processing and presenting the information by modules. It needs a trade between lack and excess of information, where the information gives the right meaning at the different phases of the organizational chain.

First it is necessary the distinction between treatment information, which supports the individualized diagnose, and the medical-tactical information that supports the resource management:

- Treatment information: information that supports the treatment of casualties. It is the individualized diagnose of each casualty that indicates the injuries or illness, and the affected body areas. This information is a reference to apply medicaments or different emergency treatments, as immobilization, amputation, hemorrhage support, etc. It is relevant for the paramedics on the field attending the victims and must be accessible at the incident area, at the transportation and the hospitals. This information is equivalent to the information recorded on the triage card.
- Medical-tactical information: information necessary to support the planning of resources. It is relevant for the senior emergency physicians, for the incident and the organizational commander. It specifies the emergency level, and it is necessary in order to know the amount of casualties and its category and the type of transportation. The logistics rely on this operation, and the information should be continually updated to take accurate decisions. This information is equivalent to the one documented in the organizational protocols and the management whiteboards, see section 2.1.3.

The collection and presentation of digital information during MCI should be simple and familiar to the emergency physicians. New systems should support the collection of treatment and medical-tactical information and present it in a clear form. Radical changes would overwhelm the health workers and would not accelerate the information flow and processing. New technologies must be intuitive and not far from the typical triage tags. They have been used for the last forty years so new technologies should not challenge the health workers. For example, active triage tags incorporating small buttons, and providing a simple human interface where paramedics should scroll through functions and fight against the poor visibility of LCD, would not be adequate for the MCI scenario.

As mentioned, a new design requires the implication of health workers experts on the management of MCI scenarios. Only in this way the conception of a suitable solution that is simple and familiar to the emergency physician's area, and that provides meaningful information can be possible.

4.1.2 User-Centered Conception Method

A sense-making approach requires an intensive interaction with end users. This section presents the results of the user-centered approach. With the objective to achieve a sense-making concept, discussion on the state of the art and research, experiences and lessons-learned took place with experts from the emergency. The new concept should be a sense-making IT platform able to abstract and organize casualty's digital information and present it in a meaningful form. The information must support the continuous planning at the incident area.

In order to support the user-centered design, a collaboration with the company antwortING and the German Red Cross took place.

Numerous interviews and workshops took place with at least six experts to conceive a new platform. Modern technologies and related projects were analyzed; it was deduced that they still not fit the requirements explained in section 3.1.3. State of the art and advantages of new ICT were as well discussed, concluding that projects from section 2 have not yet implemented them completely correct. They are not accurate enough due to the intermittent information flow, or they generate uncertainty because of the constant and meaningless alarming. Another conclusion is that health workers are overwhelmed by new and non-sense information. For example, either they have to confirm and correct automatic alerts or they even have to decide between various versions of electronic tags for the different types of casualties. The result of discussions with the experts is a set the guidelines for a new modular information technology. These guidelines are described as follows:

Guidelines for a Modular MCI Assisted-Management System

A modular concept of a sensor-assisted and mobile computer MCI Management was specified together with experts from the rescue field. In order to trace the guidelines, the main discussion points were: lessons learned from the state of art and research, the usability of sensor information and the health workers information. The role of these technologies was discussed as well. A new MCI management-system requires the coexistence of different ITC platforms, like PDAs, sensor and wireless technologies. These technologies are similar to the already presented projects, but a new approach must have a precise meaning and role for all its components. The general aim is to support the tactical planning and the medical care on-site.

The objective of the new system is to assist the decision-making at the incident area where tactical planning requires information describing and specifying the global scenario, number of casualties, categories, transport. This information is the base for the estimation of medical and transportation resources. Treatment information establishes the personalized emergency assistance, and it should be based only on the physician's criteria. Additionally, information should also be always accessible. Figure 4.3 explains the information and communication modules for the new approach.

In contrast to the existing platforms, this new modular approach is conceived to satisfy the various information necessities strategically, organizing and presenting the information to a different rescue personnel. Aside the lessons learned discussed in section 3.1.2., the guidelines for the different modules of the new approach are explained next:

Information Modularity

First of all, the implementation of a hybrid information platform is necessary. As mentioned, the collection of treatment and medical-tactical information is the primary requirement. Different information modules should respond to the multiple data necessities. Until now, no platform was able to gather sensor and manual information accurately and give a simple and standard meaning. Commanders and physicians are overwhelmed with new information forms such as alarms, long tables, physiological data and raw signal.

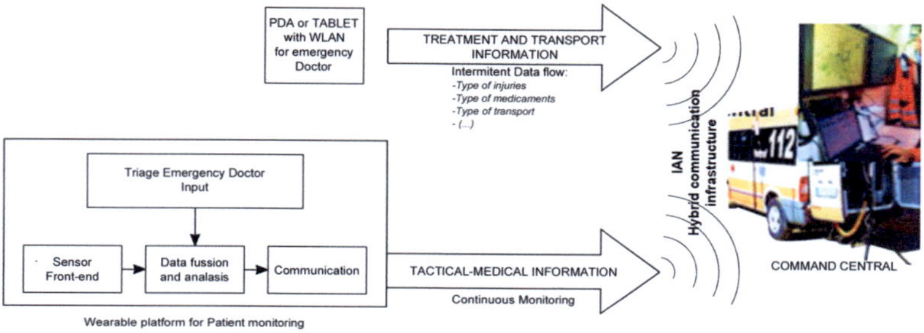

Figure 4.3: System concept to support the collection of medical-tactical information at MCIs

A new approach to take full advantage of data processing has to filter, abstract and present relevant information in a meaningful form. Only in this way, new ICT can reduce the processing effort of health workers and assist the management of the operation.

Automatic triage and diagnose are not enough precise so doctors must perform them. There is background difference, which depends on each patient; a sensor-based platform is not able to consider all the necessary context variables, and it ca not provide a reliable, specific triage or diagnose. Thus, the implementation of PDAs is still necessary to collect and organize digitally the treatment and diagnose information introduced by physicians. The triage and diagnose are significant information to provide proper health care at the treatment area. On the other side, the dynamism of the emergency scenario makes the intermittent data allocation inaccurate for the tactical planning. An accurate decision-making requires a constant overview of the patient condition on the field. Thus, an electronic monitoring of the patient condition is desired.

Sense-making Sensor Information

In contrast to the platforms implementing active triage tags and integrating physiological sensor, the information should be simple and clear. In this way, a large amount of inaccurate and high variable information would not overwhelm health workers. For example, long list of physiological values is not desired. An automatic abstraction of general triage reference and tendency might be enough to support the estimation of the operational effort.

A portable sensor platform, similarly to the triage tag, must be distributed from the beginning of the operation. In this way, the estimation of the patient condition can be tracked from the beginning of the operation allowing the commanders to estimate the emergency of the scenario, without waiting for the physicians' information. An early application of the platform allows a prompt evaluation of resources. The sensor platform assists the first triage, mainly in the chaos phase, where the incident commander requires only rough information of the patient's situation.

Assisted Treatment through Individualized Diagnose

Triage paper tags represent a basis and reference for the collection of the triage and diagnose information. It must be accessible at the triage treatment and transport area; doctors and paramedics must carry a PDAs, where they can introduce and access information. Central servers are used to store the information; with a WLAN, e.g. IEEE 802.15. network paramedics can log the information. In this way, paramedics can follow the instructions to provide the required care by only accessing the information that doctors recorded through a PDA.

Physicians must submit information similar to the triage card, as the type of injury and illness, the affected zone, medicaments and transport, as well personal information as age, name and allergies. This information also supports the commanders with the distribution of medicaments and the organization of transport in order to achieve a better-specialized treatment.

4.1.3 Continuous and Automatic Pre-Triage

The main challenge and innovation of the new platform relies on the correct use of the sensor information. Together with the experts it was decided that the sensor information should only provide a general reference of the casualty condition, in the form of pre triage. This electronic pre triage report has the advantage to indicate the tendency of the emergency; it must automatically distinguish between critical and non-critical patients. This information must regularly be updated to assist the commander from the beginning and during the operation. In this way, more certainty about the situation is provided, reducing the effort to estimate the need for resources. Even before the physician provide a more specific triage and diagnose.

The automatic pre triage report is to be performed by a portable active triage tag, integrating a sensor module and processing unit. The ordinary triage methods are the reference for the selection of the sensor platform and the definition of new algorithms for the automatic processing and analysis of the sensor information.

Sensor selection

The first triage which doctors perform at the first contact with the casualty determines and decide about its survival possibilities. If required, it is transported to the triage area, where more specific triage and diagnosis take place. In the first triage, a fundamental observation about the conscious level, as well as the respiration and circulation condition, are evaluated. Then, at the triage and treatment area, the START triage algorithm is commonly applied. For this reason, the START algorithm is the reference to select the physiological parameters to observe in the new platform, section 2.1.2 explains the START algorithm. Physicians evaluate first the walking capability, followed by the examination of the respiratory and the circulation condition and finally the conscious level.

Based on past experiences from other projects, it is observed that none project is evaluating the walking capacity. For the respiratory they are using either pulse oximeter or a cannula with an air flow meter and for the circulation state they are implementing an ECG, an NIBP meter or using as well a pulse oximeter. The application ECG might not practicable and appropriate for the scenario. Just, because it requires to remove clothes and to attach electrodes to the skin, moreover the signal quality depends on the conductivity of the skin that could be lowered by hair or dry skin. NIBP is also non-practicable since it requires a bulky inflate cuff, which inflation and deflation might no be adequate for a constant monitoring at a not calm situation. Moreover, the air pump would consume a considerable amount of energy, making it not a low-energy solution. In addition, NIBP has not proof to be an accurate indicator of the emergency of a casualty. Compare to the ECG and NIBP, the pulse oximeter represents a more suitable solution because its intuitive attachment way, additionally it can be implemented for the monitoring of the respiratory and circulation condition. Also, different measurement points are possible, as the finger, toe, earlobe and forehead, making more flexible its application.

Despite it is already a standard feature, present in many commercial devices, projects mentioned in chapter 3 with active triage tags have not yet integrated the walking control. Due to its portability and simplicity, it can be implemented in the new pre triage tag. It typically relies on a more axis acceleration sensor. An analysis of the energy in the different orthogonal axis set an indicator of the level and type of activity of the individual. The automatic waking monitoring would cover the first condition to the START algorithm.

An automatic analysis of the conscious level requires a more complex system, but portable systems are still under research. Since the walking capacity is also an indicator of the consciousness, it is defined as enough for this purpose.

Pre Triage Algorithm

The pre triage algorithm should provide a general and simple reference about the casualty's triage. It must only distinguish between critical and non-critical conditions. The platform evaluates the sensor information consistently and reports periodically the triage class: critic or non-critic, periodically. The evaluation protocol is defined based on the experience of expert emergency physicians, who are part of the user-centered design team. Similar to the START algorithm, the new algorithm for the remote pre triage of casualties evaluates the activity of the patient, the respiration and the circulation condition.

The platform integrates an activity sensor and pulse oximeter. Figure 4.4 shows the conditions to evaluate each parameter and to determine the criticality of the casualty. The most important parameter to be evaluated, from the physicians' perspective, is the breathing condition, followed by the circulation and the walking condition. In order to set a casualty as non-critic, all the parameters must fulfill the non-critic conditions. Whilst, a critical patient is defined, only if at least one of the three parameters is critical. Two algorithms are provided, one for adults and other for children. Emergency senior doctors must decide with context information if the actual scenario belongs to a child MCI or adult MCI. The pre triage decision is refined when the age of the casualty is documented.

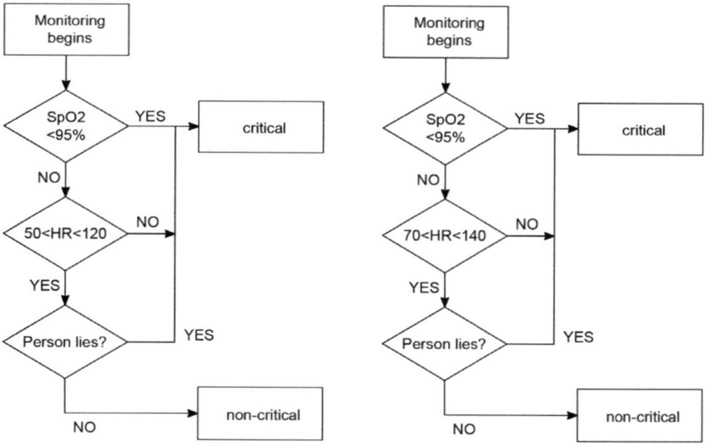

(a) Adult pre-triage (b) Child pre-triage

Figure 4.4: Diagram flow for pre-triage algorithm

4.2 Analysis of Requirements and Specification

This section discusses the requirements for the implementation of the new pre triage platform. These requirements are also a result of the user-centered design approach; multiple discussion took place in order to specify the realization principles of the new platform. The new platform must consist on a portable triage tag that should be easily attached to the patient. It must generate information to support the tactical planning of the operation, either at the commander site or on the triage and treatment areas. The tag should fulfill some technical aspects such as being uniquely identifiable to track and to relate server information to the correct patient. Moreover, the new tag similar to the triage paper cards should support the visual identification of the triage and transport situation.

4.2.1 Technical and Desing Specifications

In order to achieve a reliable system, the system must fulfill the next features: portability, manageability, and being operable, rugged, fallback prepared, identifiable and storable. Each of these technical features was specified based on the expert's experience as follows.

- *Portability:* the system should be light and should be approximately hand-size. In this way, paramedics can carry as many of these devices and attach them fast to the casualty. It should not be a bulky device that incommode the casualty.
- *Manageability:* the system should be designed in a form that the health workers can manipulate the device. Many health workers use gloves and do not have both hands-free. Human interfaces as buttons, plugs, and indicators should not challenge the health workers. They should be ergonomic conceived.
- *Operable:* Error free modular operation is required. The system should be robust against electric/electronic and mechanical errors. Buttons, plugs, indicator and communication modules should repeatedly operate correctly. The user should not be challenged to obtain the required action. The system should recognize possible errors and recover itself if not; it should indicate a failure state.
- *Rugged:* A housing should contain and protect the system. It must be ready to hard-use and unfavorable weather conditions, being prepared against humidity and water resistant. The device should resist a fall from at least one meter and should not break easily to avoid hurting the casualty or the health workers.

- *Fallback prepared:* The system must be made to provide visual information still. If a power problem occurs, the triage category must be visible. Through a mechanical interface and visual indicators, paramedics and physicians can still set and recognize the triage category. In this way, the minimum functionality of the paper triage tag is also covered.
- *Storable and ready to use:* Since MCI scenarios are not expected to occur frequently in the same area, it might be that only after a long period the devices are again in operation. Therefore, the system should be ready to operate after a long period of storage. These represent a challenge for the power modules.

4.2.2 Information Services

The new patient tag, aside from the automatic pre-triage function, should satisfy different information demands. It should assist remotely the tactical planning at the commander center and should provide a visual reference on the site to identify the patients and their triage and transport situation. These information services were as well together with the experts conceived, and they are here explained.

On-site monitoring

Similar to the paper triage cards, the new system should provide information on the field. This information comprises a visual reference for the triage category of the patient, the patient identification and also, it was decided to add an indication of the transport priority. The transport priority index should offer an indexation of critical patients, depending whether they can receive attention on the field or they can wait for hospitalization. This information should support the rapid identification and localization of patients. The emergency physician should introduce this information manually.

Triage Category

The triage categories are based on the START algorithm. Physicians must select through a rotatory switch the corresponding triage category. A colored paper label must display the type, supported by a lighting indicator.

The triage category must be visible from many meters away and many angles. The paper label provides support if a problem occurs with the lighting system.

Transport Priority

Similar to the triage category, the transport priority must through a manual switch selected. It should be also visible even if a power problem occurs. After the selection of the transport priority, the lighting triage category should blink. Transport priority should be selectable for all the triage categories. For example, in the case that a non-severe injured victim is familiar of a severely injured casualty, which has transport priority indication, the first one should belong to the same priority. In this way, paramedics recognize that they should be transported together.

Patient Identification

Patient identification should be supported by a unique ID. A QR-Code might be a solution to encode the ID. A PDA can with reader or camera can scan the QR-Code. An RFID or NFC module can support the scanning of the ID. In this way, if the paper QR-code is damaged, there is still an option to link the patient to its ID and on-line data.

System Status Indication

At last, but no less important, is the integration of a status indicator. With this indicator, the physician can identify if the device is turned on, working properly, or it has a defect. The status indicator should be a discrete lighting indicator and should not generate confusion between the other indicators. Its interpretation should be intuitive.

Remote monitoring

The new active triage tag must continuously report the casualty's information to commanders and physicians. The information must be permanently accessible through a web server application. As mentioned above, the information follows a modular principle, distinguishing between medical and tactical information. The triage tag is responsible for generating and reporting tactical information. Requirements for the remote monitoring are discussed as follows:

Medical-tactical Information

Automatic pre-triage, manual triage and transport priority belong to the tactical information relevant for the remote monitoring of the casualty. The unique new particularity is that the platform generates the pre-triage information consistently; from the moment when the tag is attached to the patient. It is decided to update this information to the central server every 30 seconds. Physicians generate manually and intermittently the diagnose and treatment information. This information should be reported together with the pre-triage information. Therefore, the information is organized at a web server application at the commander center and the physicians PDAs.

Patient Localization

In taking advantage of an electronic tag, live patient localization must be included. Patient localization provides multiple advantages since it can provide a general picture distribution of the casualties on the field. It is possible to recognize if the casualties are properly organized into the triage, treatment and transportation areas. It is also possible to identify patients with specific problems or detect the ones that are leaving the incident area. It is assumed that the majority of the rescue zones are placed outdoors. Thus, a GPS module is desired as a localization module.

An RSSI triangulation method is not desired because it requires a set of additional infrastructure to provide reference points. This approach represents an extra effort for rescuers and is not practical. RSSI triangulation might be more suitable for situations where reference nodes are already placed, such as in indoors scenarios. Since it is assumed that the first respond during MCI scenarios happens mainly outdoors, RSSI triangulation might not be a quick practicable solution.

4.2.3 Communication Services

MCI scenarios can be extended over large areas. Communication infrastructure should provide connectivity over the whole incident area. Wireless communication based on IEEE 802.15 might require many repeaters to cover an area larger than 100 m; while communication over the incident area might require connectivity over a 1000 m region.

In order to specify the communication requirements for the IAN, an extreme situation was depicted. In this scenario, the safe areas where triage, treatment and transport took place were half kilometer away from the event area. Moreover, the situation might require multiple safe areas extended over an area larger than 2.5 km2.

IEEE 802.15 hot spots for safe zones: triage, treatment and transport areas

After the first general triage occurs, casualties with surviving possibilities are transported to safe areas, where most of the first response activities take place. Triage, treatment and transport preparation occur on these areas, where physicians collect and report relevant data about the patients. Physicians are geared with PDAs able to access a web portal where to introduce or access the patient information. Wi-Fi connectivity is required over these safe zones. Since these areas are concentrated rather than expanded, IEEE 802.15 must be enough to provide the required connectivity.

Depending on technical characteristics of the incident, multiple safe areas can exist, each requiring a hotspot with Wi-Fi connectivity. Modular Wi-Fi connectivity would allow the information to reach the main server, from where commanders and physicians can log and track the information of the scenario.

Pre-Triage Broadcast over large incident areas

In order to make from the pre-triage data a valuable information, it must be available from the moment it is attached to the casualty. The pre-triage data must be reported even before the patient is transported to the safe areas. As mentioned above, depending on the technical circumstances, the command center can be placed far from the incident area, even 1000 m away. This scenario requires that the wearable triage tag connects to the main server covering large areas.

Wireless sensor network based on IEEE 802.15.4 as Zigbee can connect over 100 m in line of sight and might require a certain number of routers to allow a multi-hop communication to provide connectivity over large areas. Projects as AID-N required the set of anchor nodes on the field.

This set of field infrastructure might challenge the paramedics and might not be a practical solution.

Technologies with lower frequency bands, as Sub-1 GHz and GSM technologies, can represent a solution to cover extended large areas with low power radio modules. However, the bandwidth is affected and reduced. In order to avoid packages collision, small data packages must be intermittent transmitted.

4.3 System Concept

Based on the discussion with experts on the matter and the formulated requirements, a new concept is now introduced, and it is presented in this section. A modular conception is conceived to cover all the specified functions. In the first place, the modular architecture of the new wearable triage tag is shown, then the housing, and finally the communication and the interaction with the incident area network.

4.3.1 Wearable Casualty Monitoring Device

The new triage tag consists of an electronic wearable device. A portable and wearable platform with different electronics modules is presented. The electronics perform the multiple tasks as the acquisition of physiological signals and their processing, patient localization, and the communication of the automatic pre triage information. Also, a housing concept is introduced to support the necessary interaction with paramedics and physicians on the field. Figure 4.5 depicts the most important features of the new device.

Modular System Architecture

The modular conception of the electronic platform is divided into four main modules, pre-triage, triage, localization and communication. A host processor performs as a control unit, managing the interface between the different modules. It also analyze the various data and pack the results; it controls the transmission and analysis rate.

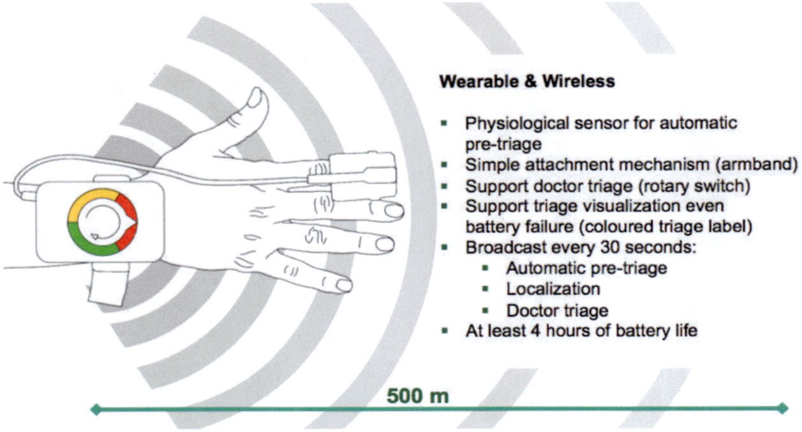

Figure 4.5: System concept for the new wearable platform for patient monitoring

The host processor acquires the data established through the human interfaces, from external buttons; in this way, the triage and transport priority are set up. A power module is necessary to handle the energy consumption and allows an operability of at least five hours.

Housing

The concept of the housing system is depicted in figure 4.5. It is conceived to support the specified requirements in the previous sections, as portability, manageability, operability, and to provide buttons interfaces where to set the triage and transport priority. It also has visible indicators to show the triage and transport categories. These visible indicators are light emitting diodes (LEDs) and physical labels; the last could still provide the triage information, even if power or electronic system problems occur.

An adjustable armband allows a simple attachment system to any type casualty, independently of age and size. Depending on the circumstance, the system can be attached to the wrist or the ankle. Both body parts

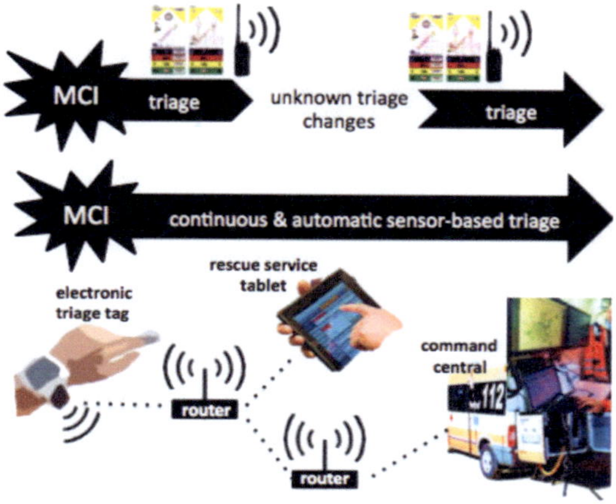

Figure 4.6: Differnces between the state of the art and the new system concept [RHG+14]

are adequate to attach a pulse oximeter probe. Finger and toes are ordinary body areas, where to measure. The proximity to the measurement areas avoids the necessity to use long cable, disturbing the treatment and management of the casualty.

4.3.2 Information Flow Process

The new wearable triage tag is a submodule, which belongs to an MCI management information and communication system. This system comprises a web portal where the commanders can track the scenario's information, PDAs where physicians collect detailed patient information and communication infrastructure to support the interaction between the different information modules. Figure 4.6 shows the interaction between the different modules and the information flow.

The triage tag automatically generates a pre-triage report, and then a web portal organizes and presents the pre-triage information and the patient localization. Information can be logged on-site from mobile computers o from desktop computers at the command center. Aside the automatic generated pre-triage information and the patient localization, the triage and transport priority are regularly communicated by the new wearable triage and monitoring tag.

Physicians, which are performing the casualty's triage and recording digitally patient information interacts in two ways with the triage tag. One is the manual selection of the triage and transport category; the other is the digital identification of the triage tag. In this way, the patient information is related to the attached triage tag. Triage and transport categories remain visible at the triage tag to support on the field the recognition of patient's situation.

Physician record personal patient information and detailed diagnosis and they also set the treatment procedures for the casualty. Later at the treatment area, paramedics and physicians can access the patient information to proceed with the patient care.

Finally a central server stores, analyzes and presents the information through a web portal. Here the information fusion from different data sources takes place. Statistics to support the tactical planning are presented to the commanders. They can follow the quantity of casualties and their triage and transport categories, and if desired, they can track detailed information of the patients situation.

4.4 Summary

Advantadges and disadvantages have been recognized in the introduction of new ICT to the MCI field. This chapter presents the conception of a novel wearable platform to overcome the lack of patient information. The new technology is necessary to plan emergencies resources from the beginning of the operation. The new platform constantly communicates an estimation of the criticaity of the victim's status. The incident officer would be able to estimate constantly the effort to clear the site.

Requirements for the development of the new platform are the result of many discussions and interviews with experts in the emergency and rescue field, including the german red cross.. Next chapter discusses the implementation of the new device.

5 Implementation of a Wearable Active Triage Tag

In the last chapter, the principles and guidelines for the implementation of a new wearable triage device are established. This chapter explains the implementation and integration process. The last chapter also depicts the different development stages. Starting with the selection of hardware modules, as physiological sensors, localization, process unit and communication. Followed by the software architecture which includes the definition of the sensor data fusion and analysis process, which performs the automatic pre-triage. In addition, the integration of processing algorithms is as well explained. Processing algorithms comprises a decision tree for the estimation of the patient activity and the parsing of localization packets. The communication routines and information packing protocols are also described.

A systematic and rapid prototyping strategy was followed. Firstly the hardware architecture and basic software functionalities were integrated into a tabletop prototype and tested a subsystem of a complete MCI Management System. Secondly, the first wearable system was integrated: with the aim to test the performance of all technical functions such as communication, localization and to get a first impression of the usability on the field. Finally, a wearable system fulfilling the technical and user requirements is presented. This last version was a miniaturization of the whole wearable triage platform, and it includes a housing with an end-product oriented design. In this way, it was possible to get a more realistic feedback about its usability during different tests.

5.1 Hardware Selection and Architecture

In the first place, the selection of the hardware modules and the architecture is described. Three main subsystems are identified in the wearable triage system. They perform the sense and acquisition of the patient data, which comprises physiological and localization data. A processing unit is responsible control all the system functionalities, to analyze the sensor information and to abstract relevant information for the triage and localization of the victim. A radio technology is presented to perform the specified communication task between the triage tag and the data management center.

5.1.1 Active Modules for Patient Monitoring

As explained in section 4.1, a continuous and automatic pre-triage and the patient localization are required to support the logistical plan of the operation. In this section, the modules to perform this task are presented and discussed.

Pre-triage Sensors: Respiration, Circulation and Activity

Section 4.1.3 discussed the conception of the pre-triage algorithm. It requires the monitoring of the respiration, circulation, and activity condition of the patient. A benchmark of different commercial solutions was conducted to support the selection of the pre-triage sensors.

Pulse Oximeter

The monitoring of the respiration and the circulation condition required the implementation of a pulse oximeter. It indicates the oxygen saturation in the blood and the heart rate. Section 2.3.2 discussed the principles around pulse oximetry.

An OEM module from the company Medlab is selected as a pulse oximeter module. Figure 5.1.1 shows the module and table 5.1.1 presents the technical specification, see $http://www.medlab-gmbh.de/$.

Size	40x20x1 mm
Weight	4 g
Operating Voltage	3.3 V DC +200 mV, -100 mV @ 15 ... 20 mA
SpO2	Measuring range: 30% ... 100 % Accuracy: 90% ... 100% : 1% 80% ... 89% : 2% 70% ... 79% : 3% below 70% : unknown
Heart rate	Measuring range: 25 ... 248 bpm Accuracy: +/- 1%
Interface	serial interface CMOS, 9600 baud, 8N1, asynchronous

Table 5.1: Technical specification

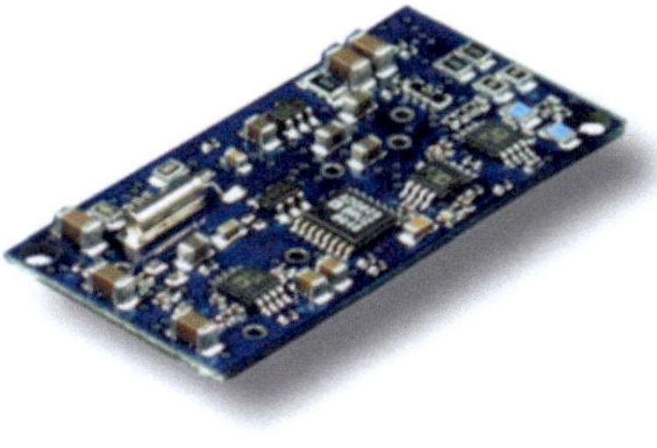

Figure 5.1: Pulse oximeter OEM module

Label - Marker byte	0xF8	0xF9	0xFA	0xFB	0xFC	
Content	Pleth wave sample points	SpO2	Hear rate	Info byte 0x00 OK 0x01 Sensos disconnected 0x02 No finger in Probe 0x03 Low perfusion 0x45 Selftest error	Quality index bit 7 to 4 Quality 0 ... 10 0 ->best quality	Perfusion index bit 3 to 0 001 perfusion <= 0.25% 010 0.25% <perfusion 0.5% 011 0.5% <perfusion 1% 010 1% <perfusion 2% 010 2% <perfusion 4% 010 4% <perfusion 8% 010 perfusion >= 8%

Table 5.2: EG000352 information protocol

The module has a UART interface and a predefined information protocol. A parser module is necessary to read the sensor information. Table 5.2 presents the data communication protocol of the sensor.

Acceleration Sensor

Acceleration sensors are typical for the monitoring of human physical activity. Acceleration signals from a two or three axis sensor are the basis for the classification of the activity. Due to its minimal size and power consumption, they are suitable for the integration of a wearable system. A three-axis sensor provides information into a three-dimensional orthogonal system, allowing a more reliable classification. Thus, it is preferred for the integration of the triage tag.

The acceleration sensor is selected taking as a reference the work presented in the previous work of Jatoba et al. [JGO$^+$08]. A MEMS triaxial acceleration sensor with an amplitude range of $\pm 6g$, resolution of 16 bits and 80 Hz of sampling frequency. An ADXL345 from Analog Devices is selected. It is a 3-axis acceleration sensor with a resolution up to 13 bits at $\pm 16g$. It allows up 3200 Hz of sampling frequency. It is a configurable module allowing information streaming at different rates and resolutions. It requires an SPI connection to control the module and to transfer the data. This module is indicated for low power applications only requiring a voltage range of 2.0 V to 3.6 V at 23 μA.

Victim Localization

As mentioned in section 3.2, triage and treatment zones are normally outdoors. Thus, victim localization with GPS technology is expected to be suitable for this scenarios. The variety of GPS modules is large. Therefore, the selection criterium is based on the integration of a wearable device. A module with an integrated antenna with an accuracy of minimum five meters is necessary, and it must be low power consumption specified.

As a result of the benchmark of different modules, the UP501 from Ublox is selected. Table 5.3 presents the technical characteristics of the modules.

Size	22x22x8 mm
Weight	9 g
Voltage operation	3.0 to 4.2 V @ 75 mW
Position accurarcy	2.5 m
Time to first fix	Cold start: 34 s Warm start: 34 s Hot start: 1 s
Antenna	Embedded 18 mm patch antenna
Interface	UART 9600 Baud CMOS level NMEA Protocol

Table 5.3: UP501 Technical characteristics

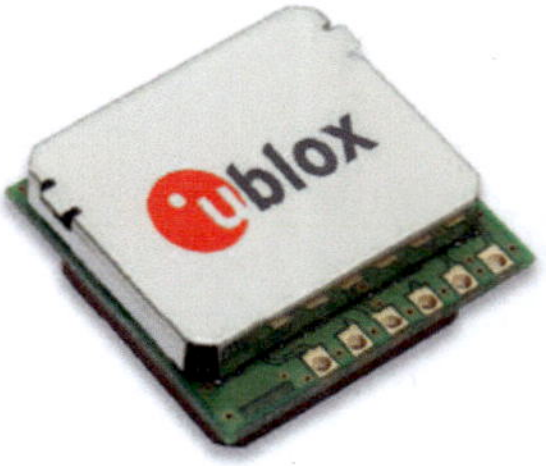

Figure 5.2: Ublox GPS OEM module UP501

The relevance of the UP501 module is its low power consumption char-acteristics and its low fist time to fix.

Also it can establishes a fast first contact with the satellites: between 1 to 40 seconds, see also *http://www.ublox.com*.

5.1.2 Data Processing and Communication Unit

The combination of controller and a radio module performs the information processing and communication tasks. A micro-controller is specified as the processing unit of the wearable platform. It must provide enough interfaces for the sensor and localization units. Also, connection flexibility to test different modules for the rest of the functionalities, such as the lighting triage visualization system and the input triage system. The selection of the radio module was performed together with experts from the company IMST, developer and provider of radio technologies.

Processing Unit MSP430F5438

The micro-controller selected as processing and control unit is the MSP430 F5438. The architecture of the micro-controller offers the required flexibility, multiple types of ports and interfaces that permit the integration of different approaches for all the required modules. It is suitable for ultra-low-power applications. Thus, it is adequate for the integration into portable and wireless systems. The processing characteristics also enable flexibility to implement diverse and complex processing as classification algorithms for the analysis of sensor data.

The following characteristics are some relevant technical aspects of the selected micro-controller. The system frequency can be set up till to 25 MHz, providing sufficient computing power for the data processing for multiple sources. This module is a 16 bit RISC structure basis, supporting standard data lengths in programming. A Hardware multiplier is available, and 32 bit operations are supported. Three different 16 bit timers are disposable: TA0, TA1, and TB0. They support parallel routines for the controlling of multiple external units and the handling of interrupted events. Different configurable interfaces are available, including the required serial connections: 2 different USCI modules are present: USCIA for UART, SPI and I2C and USCIB for SPI. 256 kB of flash memory supports to scale the complexity of the data processing algorithms. The operation of the device requires a low voltage supply from 1.8 V to 3.6 V and a low power consumption of 230 μA. Moreover, various low power modes allow further software configuration for energy saving, e.g. by calling a standby mode. It also has 87 GPIO pins that support the testability of different concepts for the lighting and input triage systems. Figure 5.3 shows the functional architecture of the micro-controller.

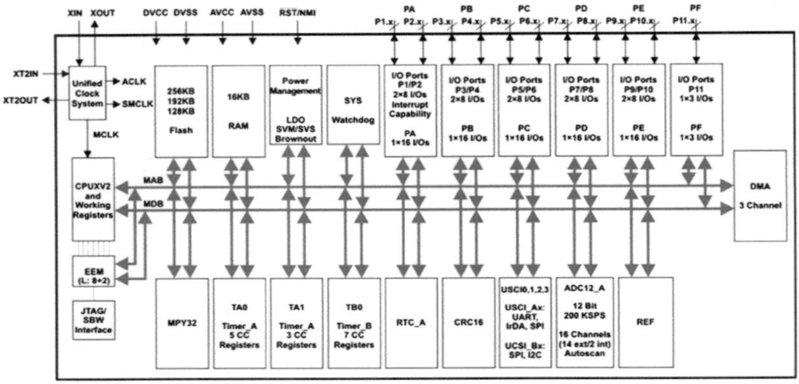

Figure 5.3: MSP430F5438A functional arquitecture (http://www.ti.com)

Radio Module sub-1 GHz

Communication between the wearable triage tag and the data center must cover a radius of at least 500 m large. The introduction of low power radio modules in the sub-1 GHz bands enables the large range communication. A new WLAN standard, the IEEE 802.11.ah based on sub-1 GHz bands is being prepared and planned for 2016 [cite]. Sub-1 GHz technologies represent an advantage over IEEE 802.15.4 technologies. Sub-1 GHz technologies, compared to conventional WLANs protocols operating at 2.4 GHz, improve the transmission ranges and ensure communication over longer links with the cost of bandwidth [cite]. Sub-1 GHz radio communication is suitable for multiple applications such as sensor networks [cite], automatic meter reading, industrial monitoring and control, and building automation.

A Sub-1 GHz technology from the partner company IMST is the radio communication module for the new triage communication platform. It works in the bands: 868 MHz and 169 MHz. Figure 5.1.2 shows the module and table 5.4 presents its technical characteristics; information is IMST portal: http://www.imst.com.

Size	20x25x5 mm
Voltage operation	2.3 to 3.6 V @ typ. 40 mA Tx
RF Range	1 to 2 km @ 169 MHz 6 to 7 km @ 868 Mhz
Antenna	Dipole with 2 dBi for Tx 35x46 mm @ 868 MHz 20x40 mm @ 169 MHz
Interface	UART

Table 5.4: RF module technical characteristics

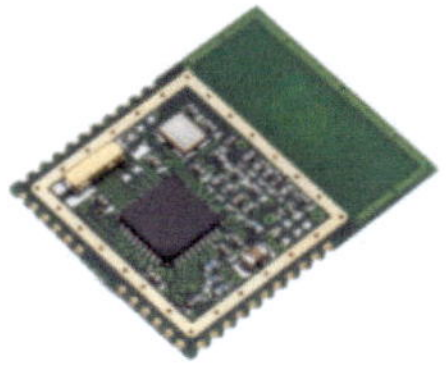

Figure 5.4: IMST RF module

5.1.3 Hardware Architecture and Power Specification

In the last section, technical characteristics of hardware modules performing data sensing, fusion, analysis and communication were presented. These technologies represent the basic hardware architecture for the new triage tag. Based on the interface properties, the general system architecture is presented in figure 5.5. The free ports of the micro-controller remain available to test different approaches for the manual introduction and visualization of the triage category.

In the last descriptions of the hardware modules, the power specifications were as well included. Taking into consideration the five hours requirement of a continuous operation, a power source of at least 3.3 V @ approx 500 mAh is necessary. Sections 5.2.2 and 5.2.3 present different power solutions for the different prototypes and include as well the power requirements for the triage category LEDs.

5.2 Software Modules and Functions

In this section, the software integration is described. The main software functions comprise the acquisition, processing, analysis and the communication routines. The wearable tag must provide the pre-triage class, the localization, and the triage information. The pre-triage information is based on data from the OEM pulse oximeter and the acceleration sensor. The localization information is provided by an OEM GPS, and the triage is a manual entry. The system is extended with memory to support the fallback requirements. In this way, the information is not lost if battery change is necessary.

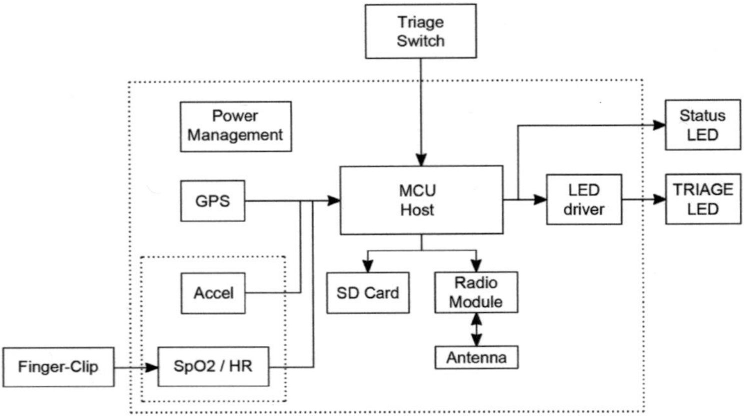

Figure 5.5: Hardware architecture

Parsing routines are necessary for the interpretation of data from the OEM modules. Statistical analysis functions and machine learning mechanisms are necessary for the classification of the sensor data. Interrupters must be configured to detect manual entry; a protocol is the base for the data communication structure. Configuration and control functions are necessary to communicate the different modules with the host controller. These functions, together with the routines and the software architecture, are described in detail in this section.

5.2.1 Patient Classification - Automatic Triage Report

In the first place, the routines to parse and analyze the sensor information for the estimation of the pre-triage are described. The requirement is to report every thirty seconds an estimation regarding the patient's condition. The system must recognize between two classes: critic and non-critic. Section 4.1.3 discussed the new pre-triage algorithm.

The pre-triage classification requires the support of two hardware modules, a pulse oximeter, and an acceleration sensor. The pulse oximeter provides, with a rate of approximately one second, information about the oxygen saturation and the heart rate. Only a parsing function is necessary to read the data. In the case of the acceleration sensor, a more complex processing routine is necessary to identify the activity or position. The parsing and processing routines for both sensor information are explained as follows.

Pulse Oximeter

The EG000352 module from Medlab provides an unsynchronized update from the oxygen saturation (SpO2) and the heart rate. The information update rate is approximately one second. The module is a unidirectional communication device. After the power up, the module starts to transmit data to the host without any needs for commands or another setup. The SpO2 value, the pulse rate, the plethysmographic curve and several status bytes are transmitted. The interface configuration needed is the UART with 9600 baud rate and a standard protocol, which are explained in the respective technical manual [thesis] [Medlab Manual].

The parsing function follows the labels structure of the module's protocol, see table 2.15(b). The SpO2 and heart rate are saved into a buffer approximately each second. After thirty seconds, the mean of each one is calculated and used in the automatic in the pre-triage algorithm.

Acceleration Information

The pre-triage algorithm also requires the classification of the activity and position of the patient. A 3-axis acceleration sensor is used for this purpose. As mentioned above, a more complex processing algorithm is necessary. The ADXL345 uses four wires for communication with the microcontroller. From the microcontroller configuration perspective, it is a 3-wire SPI communication with an extra connection pin, CS (chip select). The CS is used to set the slave (accelerometer) mode active and ready to start exchanging information.

The implementation of read and write functions follows in the definition of the Sparkfun Quickstart Guide [cite]. The initialization routine comprises the activation of the SPI port, followed by a configuration routine, where all necessary registers to define the data rate and format are set up. The selected configuration was +/8 g, 10-bit resolution, which, according to the datasheet of the sensor, is approximately 64 LSBs per g value. In order to read from memory registers containing the acceleration values for each axis x, y and z, a read function is called. It sends the address of the respective registers and reads the answer back from the ADXL345. The SPI interface works on the basis of bytes. Therefore, all of the functions described, demanding communication directly with the device, use sub-routines to send and receive each byte individually.

The sensor information is generated for each axis at 64 Hz, a buffer for each axis is necessary to store the information, and an automatic activity classifier is to be trained. Next section explains the implementation of the classification algorithm.

Activity Classification Algorithm Implementation and Verification

The algorithm and training system is taken from the previous work reported by Jatoba et al.[JGO$^+$08, JGK$^+$08]. The classifier is a decision tree approach that takes into account the absolute energy and the direction of the energy vectors. The basis for estimation of the intensity of the activity is the energy expenditure *EEAC*, calculated from the acceleration data from each axis a_x, a_y and a_z. If EEAC is greater than a precalibrated non-active threshold, the patient would be walking, else the orientation of the acceleration vector a_y is used to determine the position of the patient:

$$\cos\beta = \frac{a_y}{EEAC} \text{ where EEAC} = \sqrt{a_x^2 + a_y^2 + a_z^2} \quad (5.1)$$

$$\beta = 180^\circ \pm 40^\circ \rightarrow sittingorstanding \quad (5.2)$$

$$\beta \neq 180^\circ \pm 40^\circ \rightarrow lying \quad (5.3)$$

The development of the activity classification algorithm is divided into two steps. First, a classification tree is trained in Matlab. Ten hours of acceleration data of an accelerometer attached to the wrist of ten different individuals are used as a reference. The half of the dataset is used for training and the rest for verification. Different combinations of data sets are used for the training of the decision tree. Figure 5.7 presents an example of the classification process.

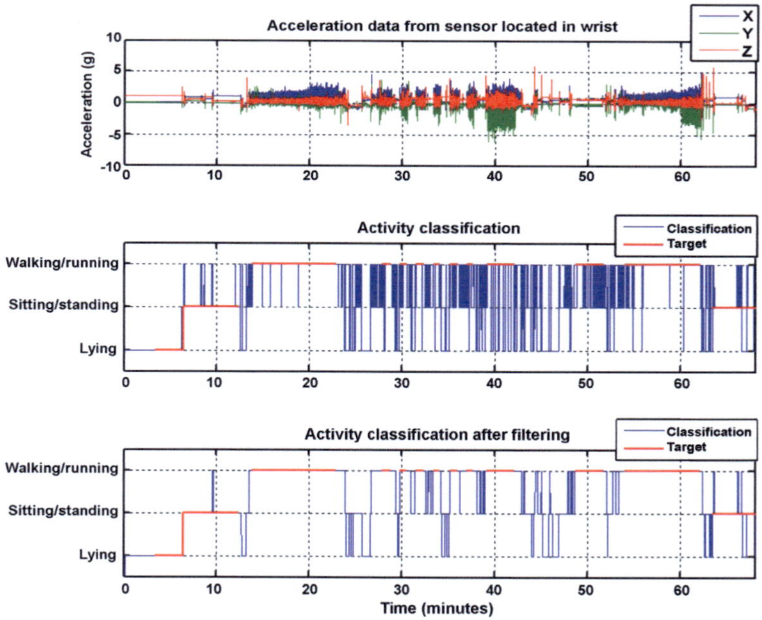

Figure 5.6: Activity classification

The second implementation step was to generate the embedded code of the decision tree. In Matlab, the C code of the decision tree was automatically implemented. The C code was transformed into a MEX file, which is the equivalent function of a C code for Matlab. An EKGMove from the company Movisens was used, which has the same accelerometer. Sensor data was saved for different positions and activities, see figure 5.7; and classified offline in Matlab, table Tableaccres shows the results obtained.

Table 5.5: Activity classification results

		Target Class		
		lying	*siting*	*walking*
Observed Class	*lying*	1373	34	43
	siting	265	2551	109
	walking	36	193	6433
Accuracy		**93.84%**		

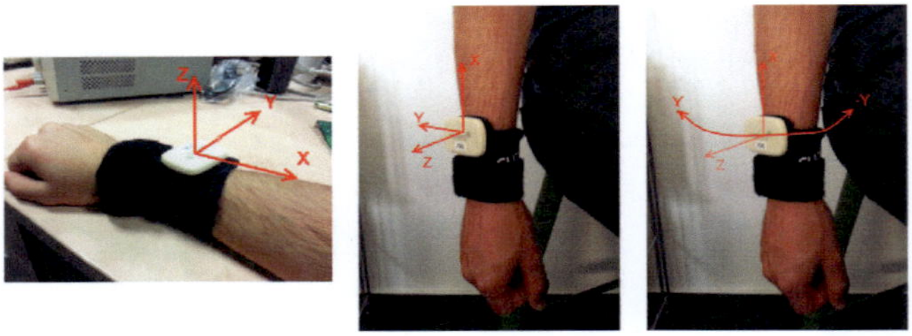

Figure 5.7: Activity data collection

Pre-Triage Algorithm Integration

Section 4.1.3 explains the pre-triage algorithm and figure 4.4 shows it. The algorithm requires the SpO2 and heart rate information as a reference of the situation of the respiration and circulation system. It requires the acceleration data as a reference for the activity. After the parsing and processing of sensor information, the fusion of all sensor data is also required. A buffer store the data for a period of thirty seconds, then, the mean value for each parameter is calculated. The mean value resulting from a period of thirty second is used to estimate whether the patient is critical or non-critic.

It is important to emphasize that the information about the pre-triage is only available to commanders, and it does not substitute the triage process. The pre-triage only indicates the tendency of the gravity and the emergency of the whole scenario, indicating the number of critical or non-critical patients in real time. This information is conceived to balance the supply of resources at the field.

5.2.2 Localization

The GPS receiver module, UP501, provides the NMEA sentences, which are the standard information protocol used by all GPS receivers. GPS receiver communication is part of the specification of the new platform. Most computer programs that provide real-time position information understand and expect data to be in NMEA format. NMEA includes the complete PVT (position, velocity, time) data computed by the GPS receiver.

The NMEA protocol contains information lines called sentences, which are completely self-contained and independent from other sentences. The sentences begin with a $ symbol, and a return/line terminates the sentences. Sentences are no longer than 80 characters. The data format is ASCII based, and commas separate each data item. Data items or variables may vary in precision, for example, the time information is expressed in decimal parts of a second, or location may have 3 or 4 decimal digits of precision. The checksum is at the end of the sentences, which will support the verification of the read data functions.

The most significant NMEA sentences for the victim localization are:

- provides essential 3D position fix data (latitude, longitude and altitude). It also includes the current time in UTC format that supports the data synchronization.
- RMC: provides essential GPS data. Compared to the GCA, it also contains velocity information.
- GSA: This sentence provides details on the type of satellite fix (cold, warm or hot). It includes the number of visible satellites and the DOP information, which is a unitless reference of the accuracy of the information. Low DOP values refer for a more accurate localization. For example, in the case of 3D fixes with four visible satellite, 1.0 DOP will be the best possible localization while other constellations can provide values even lower than 1.0.

The UP501 GPS module requires a 9600 baud rate UART communication port. As soon as the module is active, it will start to estimate the position and to stream the NMEA sentences. A parsing function is required to parse the required NMEA sentences and to interpret the data. The parser design is from in the work presented in [CdAG13]. It is a state machine which is continuously looking for the expected sentences, and when a sentence is detected, the state change to the processing of the NMEA sentence.

The GPS data is stored and reported together with pre-triage information. The next section explains into detail the communication protocol.

5.2.3 System Integration

In this section, the main routine is explained. It consists of a state machine. The main program includes all routines to configure the hardware interfaces, as well to collect and to parse the data from all modules and the routine to build the communication packages and to trigger the radio communication process.

In figure 5.8, the diagram flow is depicted. In the first state, the system initialization, interfaces and external modules configuration take place. In the second state, the system enters into a loop routine that processes, analyzes and integrates the information to be stored and communicated. An interrupt set the timing references for thirty seconds period to process sensor data and communicate the localization and condition of the patient.

Triage and Transport Information

As explained before, physicians must introduce the triage category into the wearable tag. A coded switch is the interface to set both values. When the triage category or the transport information change, an interrupt in the micro-controller triggers the process to store the new value into the triage or transport variables. Triage and transport categories should be represented for the next categories: CAT I, CAT II with transport priority, CAT II, CAT II with transport priority, CAT III, CAT III with transport priority, CAT IV and expectant.

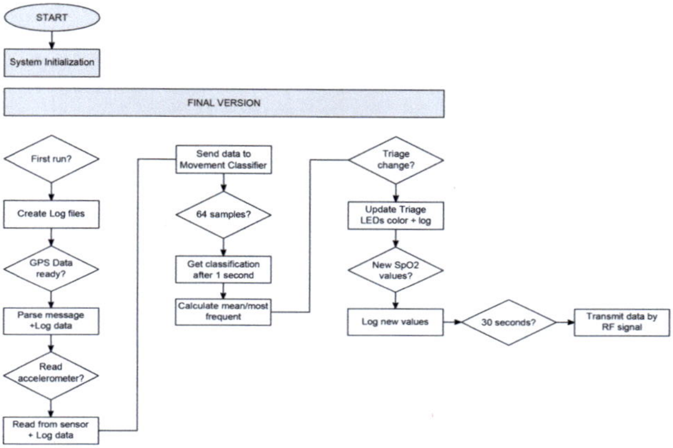

(a) Main routine algorithm

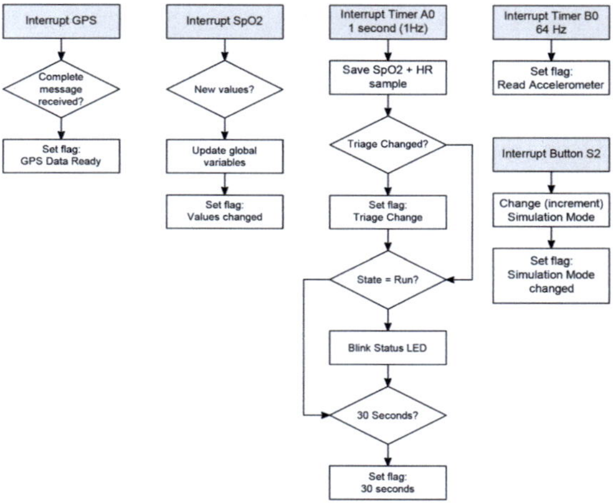

(b) Interrupt architecture

Figure 5.8: Diagram flow main routine and interrupts [CdAG13]

Storage System

As mentioned, storage capabilities are added to the system. An SD card is integrated to add flash memory. All the patient information is stored, it can be recovered, and used for experimental purposes. The writing functions require an SPI communication between the SD card and the micro-controller. A FATFS file system is implemented as in [CdAG13]. It is a generic FAT file system module for embedded systems. It is an open source software written in compliance with ANSI C, independent of hardware architecture.

The sub-routine to write information on the SD card requires first an initialization object, where the FATFS system is mounted on the card. Then a file object to write the information and finally the file must be closed.

Communication Protocol

Figure 5.9 shows the communication stack between the host controller and the radio frequency module. At the application layer, all the above-described functions are performed. A communication function will trigger the interaction with the RF module. The packet transmission works by sending the HC messages over the UART interface at 576000 bps, 8 data bits, a no parity bit and one stop bit. A serial communication protocol that comprises a series of messages with the patient information is necessary to exchange information. Figure 5.9(a) presents the message content. The message begins with the SOF, start of frame, used to label the beginning of the octet stream. It is followed by a header and payload fields, and ended with a checksum value.

The payload field contains the patient information, which should be parsed and presented at the commander portal. Figure 5.9(b) shows the structure of the payload field. The PLIFlag indicates the informa-tion referred to a certain patient and contains the hard-coded identifica-tion number. It is followed by the triage and transport category, that the emergency doctor introduced manually. Then, the pre-triage information is provided for the adult and children cases, and the status of each physiological parameters is provided as well. In the end, the localization coordinates are indicated. The GCA NMEA is packaged and compressed as figure 5.9(c) shows.

The communication between the micro-controller and the radio mod-ule is triggered based on a thirty seconds timer. Then the information is transmitted to the commander with the same rate.

SOF	Message Header Field	Playload Field	FCS
8 Bit	24 Bit	n * 8 Bit	16 Bit

(a) Message general strucutre

PLIFlag	Triage Category & Tansport Priority	Sensor Value Tendencies	Position (GPS)
8 Bit	8 Bit	8 Bit	8 Bit

(b) Payload information

1 Byte	4 Byte	4 Byte	1 Byte
BV 0: 0 – N 1 – S BV 1: 0 – E 1 - W	xm.dd X = 0 – 90 ° M = 0 – 60 min Dd = 0 – 9999	ym.dd Y = 0 – 180° M = 0 -60 min Dd = 0 - 9999	QI

xxmm.dddd: Latitude: xx = minutes: dddd= decimal part of minutes
yyymm.dddd: Longitude: yyy = degrees; mm minutes; dddd= decimal part of minutes

(c) Localization information GPS-GGA

Figure 5.9: RF communication stack

5.3 Wearable System Prototyping

This section explains the implementation process of the new wearable system. First, the technical integration of commercial development kits was performed. In this way, the interface configuration and the communication between all the modules and the host micro-controller were calibrated and tested. Simple data transfer functions were implemented to test the module's timer, the data synchronization and the radio communication.

After the implementation of the basic routines and functionalities, the design and implementation of a portable device are performed. The requirements explained in section 4.2 are taken into consideration. In the first place, the embedded platform is integrated to test the portability and usability of the device firstly, and then the radio and localization functions.

The first integration of a wearable prototype was tested and discussed with end-users and experts from the rescue and emergency field. Based on their feedback, an optimization iteration was performed. As a result, a second prototype was as well integrated and tested. The second prototype is discussed as well in this section.

The implementation of the wearable triage tag followed a rapid prototyping approach where the housing design was supported by experts in mechanical design. The prototyping steps and the different objectives are:

- Tabletop prototype: first integration with development kits, interface configuration between modules and test of the sensors, localization and communication modules.
- First portable realization: development of a printed board circuit (PCB) and integration into a housing. First tests in recreated MCI.
- Prototype optimization: technical and housing design optimization. Second test in recreated MCI.

5.3.1 Tabletop Prototyp: Basic Functions

As mentioned, the first prototyping step comprises the integration of the low-level functionalities: interface configuration, calibration and test of the data transfer. The start development kits of the different modules are under consideration. Also, for the manual set of the triage and transport categories, a rotary switch is selected. The display of the triage and transport category required the integration of the LED indicator system. Four RGB LEDs were set and controlled by TLC59711 from TI . In figure 5.10(a) it is possible to identify the rotary switch and the led system.

The main objective of the tabletop integration was to validate the parsing and communication of different data, as the pulse oximeter, localization, and pre-triage. The validation occurred during a tabletop evaluation where this first prototype interacted with the commander portal. At the time of the evaluation, it was required to run all mentioned basic functions (GPS, triage input and visualization, pulse oximeter sensor and RF communication). The RF module communicates over the 169 MHz band. Figure 5.10 shows a picture of the tabletop prototype and its evaluation.

The main program, still in an early version, had the necessary functions and routines to broadcast patient information. It included as well the reception and parsing of GPS coordinates, reading of triage switch input, set LEDs colors and mode, and finally, the RF transmission.

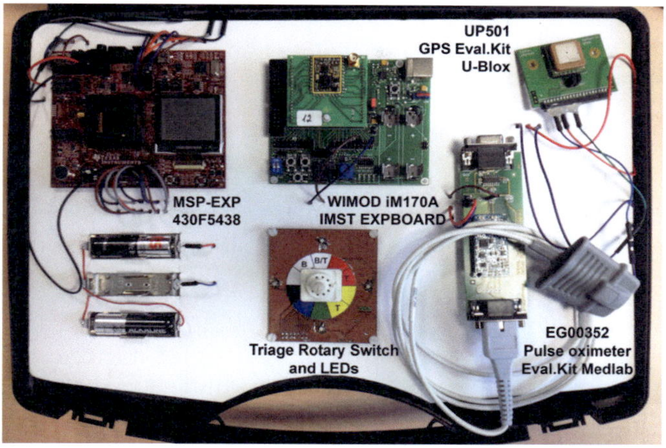

(a) Tabletop prototype

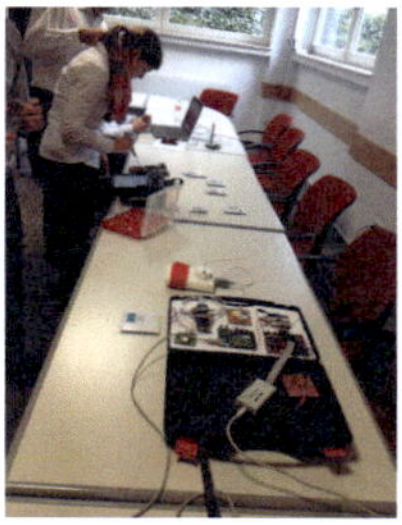

(b) Interaction with the table top prototype

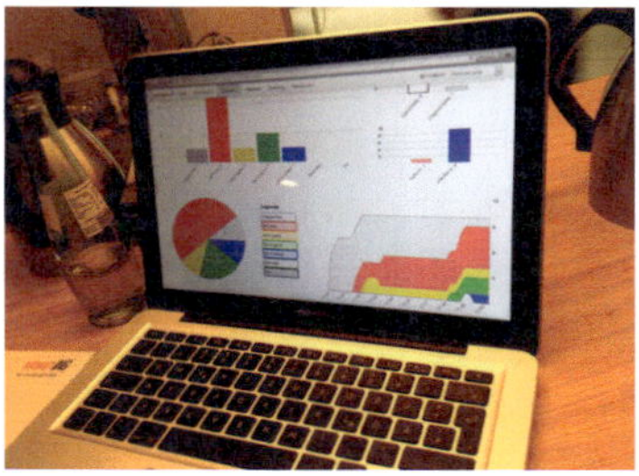

(c) Data visualization

Figure 5.10: Tabletop integration and test

During the evaluation, see figure 5.10(b), the data transmitted was verified at the commander portal, verifying in this way that the transmission was correctly performed. The expected data was then displayed, see figure 5.10(c).

Processor in the loop test-bench: Pre-Triage Routine Validation

In the first stage of hardware and sensor integration, a processor in the loop (PIL) test bench was implemented to verify the performance of the pre-triage algorithm. The test bench allowed to check the correct functionality of the classification of sensor data on the microcontroller and investigate further approaches. Figure 5.11(a) depicts the platform approach.

Table 5.6: Simulated patient cases for processor in the loop test

Simulated Patient Condition	Case 1	Case 2	Case 3	Case 4	Case 5	Case 6	Case 7	Case 8
SpO2	Ok	nOK	nOK	nOK	Ok	nOk	Ok	Ok
HR	Ok	Ok	Ok	nOk	nOk	nOk	Ok	nOk
Activity	Yes	Yes	No	No	Yes	Yes	No	No
Expected Class	non-critical	critical	critical	critical	critical	critical	critical	critical

The advantage of the tool is the ability to analyze the performance of uCs to perform the pre-triage algorithm. Different patient dummy data sets were created to represent different patient cases, depicted in table 5.6. The data was streamed to the microcontroller, in the same way, that the pulse oximeter and the accelerometer do. The microcontroller replied every thirty seconds with the pre-triage class. The PIL testbench was implemented in Matlab and Simulink.

After few corrections, the microcontroller achieved to reply always with the corresponding class, confirming the correct integration of the pre-triage algorithms. Figure 5.11(b) shows examples of these results. The system worked with simulated and real sensor data. The system shows for simulated sensor data an accuracy of 100% and for the test with real sensor data 96% of accuracy. The test supported the evaluation of the quality and reliability of the developed software routines.

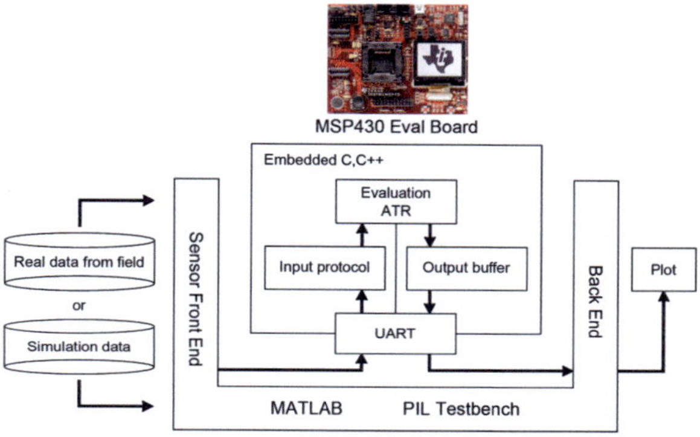

(a) PIL testbench

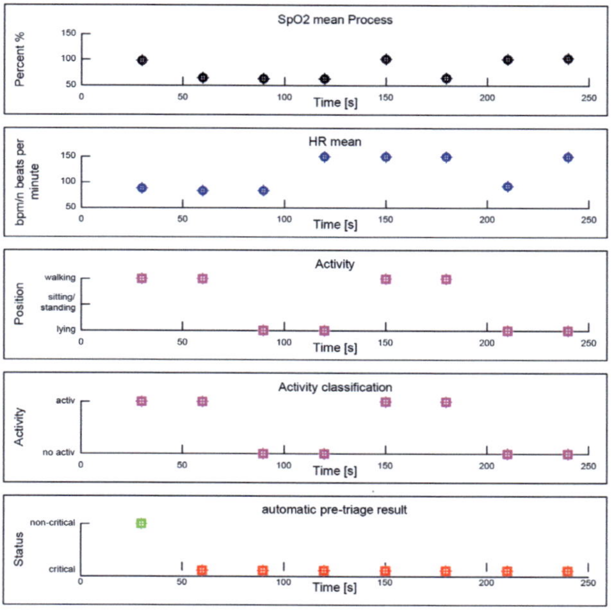

(b) PIL results

Figure 5.11: Processor in the loop testbench [Sob13]

5.3.2 Embedded Integration of the Wearable Triage Tag

After the verification of the software architecture and the technical integration of the different hardware modules, the next step is the embedded implementation of the wearable tag. The main objective of this first integration was to achieve a miniaturization of the platform. Also, to fulfill technical requirements such as the long-range communication, five meters accurate communication, five hours of battery life, real-time pre-triage and robust housing system.

The implementation of wearable tag requires the development of a PCB, a power management solution, the design of the antenna, a display system rotary triage switch and the design of the housing system. Section 4.2 discusses development criteria and systems requirements for a new platform. The design and specification for the development of the different modules are explained next.

PCB, Housing and Technical Specification

Figure 5.12 shows the PCB layout and its implementation. In the first step, a general miniaturization of the system took place. However, the size of the antenna had constrained the overall size reduction. In this first implementation was to leave space for an antenna able to reach the requirements.

Power Supply Design and Turn On System

The power requirements were constrained by the specification and consumption of each module. The table shows the power characteristics of each module. The objective was to achieve 3.3 V @ 800 mAh. A simple solution was selected in the first place; it comprised three AA alkaline batteries, and the voltage was rectified by a linear regulator. The system achieved a constant operation up to eight hours, as observed in figure 5.13. The batteries were discharged with the system operating in full mode.

The concept "remove-before-flight" was implemented as turn on mechanism of the system. A plastic ribbon between the batteries and the contact was placed. Paramedics had to pull it to turn on the tag. In this way, the system could not turn off by accident.

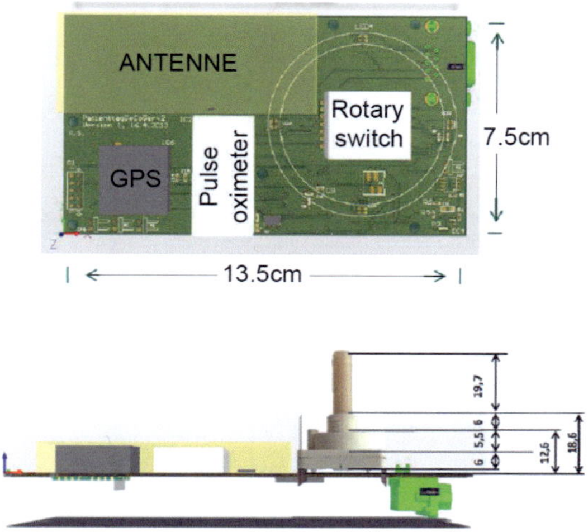

(a) PCB 3D layout

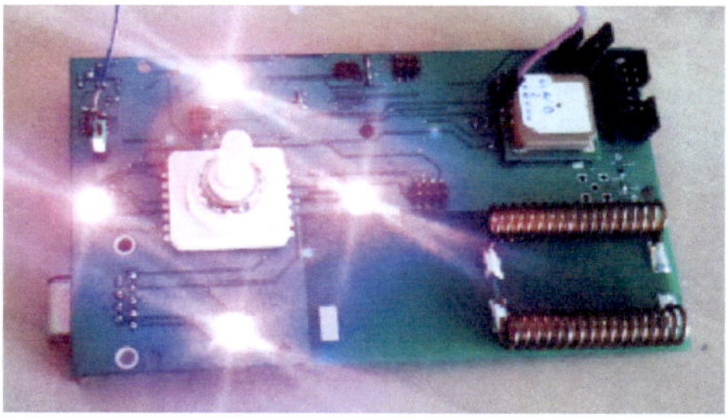

(b) PCB realization

Figure 5.12: PCB first waerable prototype

RF Modul Antenna

The RF module integration is a critical feature of the wearable device; the long range coverage requirement compromises the miniaturization of the device. The antenna design was a typical dipole with about 2 dBi gain. However, the antenna performed with 10% of efficiency since the size of the antenna was about 20 x 40 mm. The system achieved to cover a distance of 1 km.

Table 5.7: Power consumption by module

Component	Company	Part number	Typ current [mA]	Peak current [mA]
Pulse oximeter	MedLab	EG00352	15	20
GPS	Ublox	UP501	25	38
ACC	Analog Devices	ADXL345	0.14	0.14
RF-Modul	IMST		42	140
uC + SD card	Texas Instruments	MSP430F5438A	20	95
RGB LEDs x 4			216	540
		Total	**approx. 300**	**830**

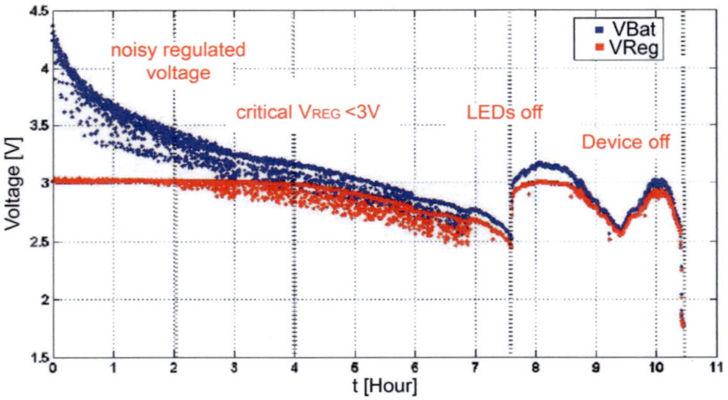

Figure 5.13: Discharge curve first wearable prototype [Sob13]

Triage Indicator

A light guide material in the form of a ring was designed, see figure 5.14(a). In this way, the color was visible from multiple directions. Around the light indicator, a label was placed to satisfy the fallback requirement. In the case of electrical failure, the system could still show the triage category.

Housing

The housing design and development was supported by a specialist designer. In this first prototype, the size is not the main priority. The development pursuit to be robust, usable and easy to manipulate. The housing design took into consideration the extreme and hard use conditions. The housing system had the objective to be intuitive and easy to use and not to challenge the paramedics. Relevant is the design of the mechanical interface for the rotary switch, as it allows an easy way to set the triage and transport category. The housing supports all the necessary interfaces, for pulse oximeter figure probe and the visualization of the triage, category, and module state. The housing was produced with a 3D printer. Figure 5.14(c) presents the housing system.

System Validation

Ten units were built and tested during MCI simulations; test methodologies and results are presented in the next chapter; feedback about the usability of the system was obtained from experts and end users. The system was optimized based on this feedback. Next section discusses the improvement iteration.

5.3.3 Prototype Optimization

Based on the evaluation and the gotten feedback from paramedics about the first prototype implementation, different optimization aspects were specified. In the first place, a size and weight reduction was necessary. A reduction in size and weight constrained the first antenna design and the use of three AA batteries as power source considerably. In second place, an optimization of the antenna was also necessary. It was observed in the first prototype that on non-line of sight (NLOS) scenarios, the distance coverage was considerably reduced. Changes in the housing are also necessary, a neutral color was required to avoid confusion on the field. The modifications for the optimization of the wearable are explained next. This optimization pursued the development of a prototype with an end-product oriented design and characteristics.

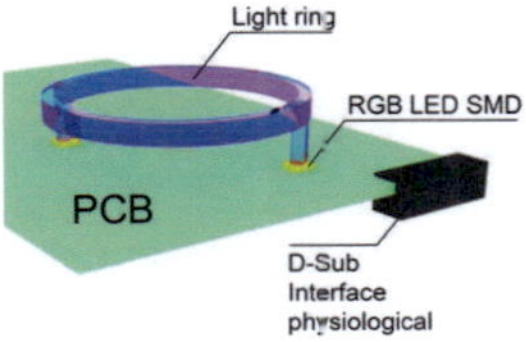

(a) Ligthing ring concept

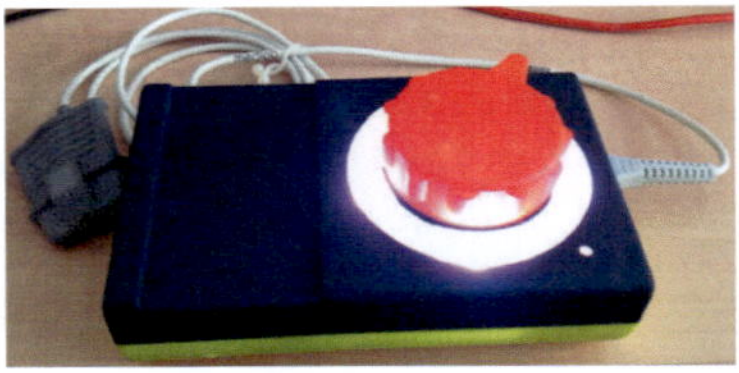

(b) Housing realization

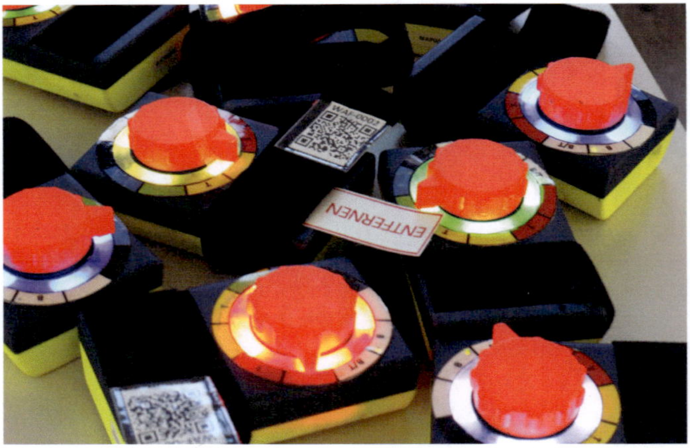

(c) Housing realization

Figure 5.14: Housing and lighting system - first wearable prototype

Power Supply Design and Turn On System

The three AA batteries were replaced by a Li-Ion accumulator. The substitution represented different advantages such as space reduction for the power system, weight reduction and the possibility to recharge the device. In this prototype, a step down/step-up converter (buck-boost) TPS63000 from Texas Instruments supported the regulation of the 3.3 V source.

The power system was tested again; figure 5.15 shows the discharge voltage curve. In comparison with the first version, the life duration was longer, and the voltage regulator provided a cleaner voltage output.

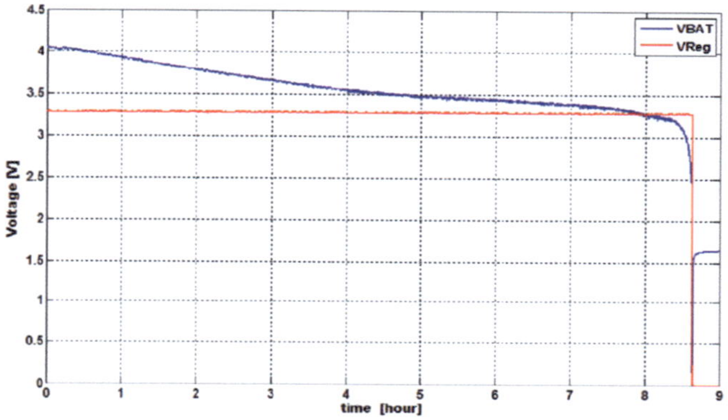

Figure 5.15: Discharge curve wearable prototype

PCB Layout & Housing

A new layout was required to miniaturize the system and improve the portability. Based on the presented modification, the new PCB was developed, figure 5.16 present the new PCB. The size was 65% reduced and the weight 56%. In addition, a new housing system was designed for the new PCB; figure 5.16(a) presents it.

The new rotary cap is designed only to show the actual triage category. In this way, it was faster to recognize the triage category visually. Following the recommendations of the experts, a neutral color was selected. A black housing was selected to improve the contrast with the color of the triage category. The armband attachment system was kept, as well as the QR-Code and the near field communication (NFC) chip for the patient identification. Figure 5.17 presents the new housing. This version housing was produced with 3D printing as the first version.

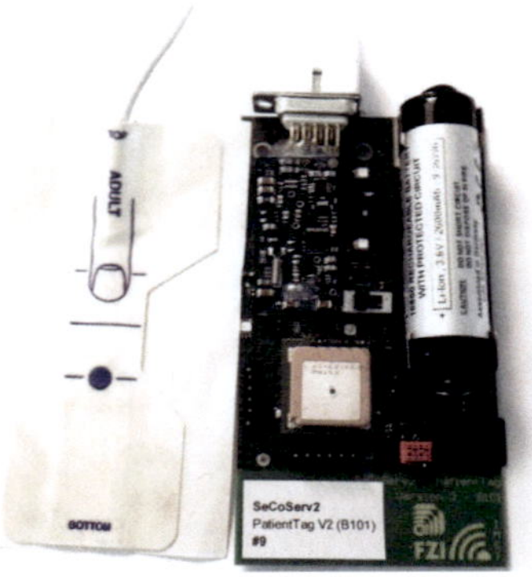

(a) PCB top view

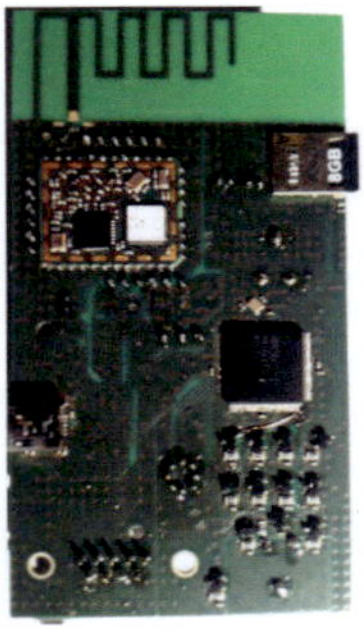

(b) PCB bottom view

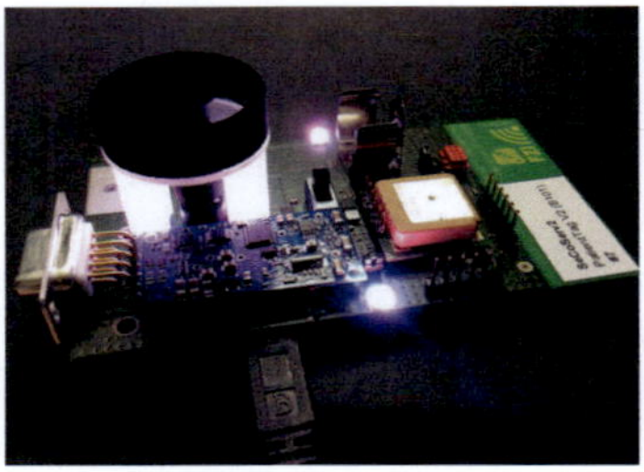

(c) PCB subsystem test

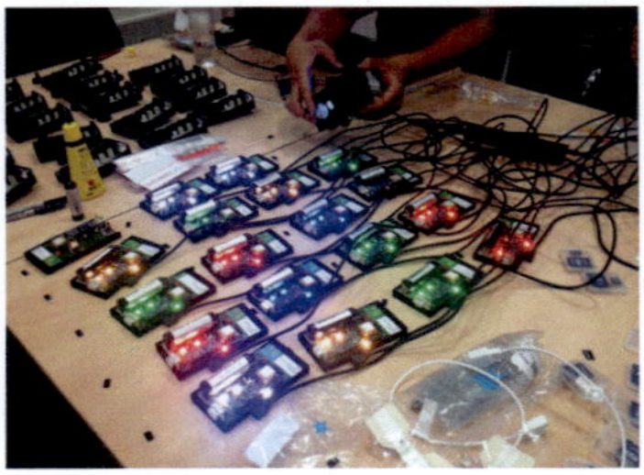

(d) PCB functional test

Figure 5.16: PCB realization for the second prototype

RF Modul Antenna

The RF module was also modified. In the new prototype, an 868 MHz module from IMST was selected, and a strip antenna was integrated. The new antenna required less space that in the first prototype, and the weight was also reduced. By 20 dBm gain, the antenna had an efficiency of 40-50%: this improvement relied on the better layout of the circuit, and the antenna was significantly larger than the wavelength. The new system was able to cover distances up to 3 km in the line of sight scenarios, representing an improvement of three times the range of the first version. Figure 5.16(b) presents the new antenna.

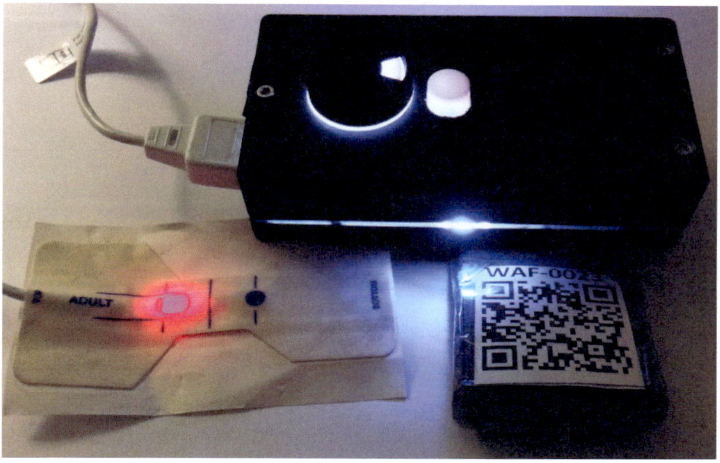

Figure 5.17: Optimized wearable platform

Selection and Indication of Triage and Transport Category

One clear option to reduce the size of the tag was the replacement of the rotary switch. It was s replaced by a mini rotary switch. In the new tag, two switches were required, one rotary to select the triage category and one slide switch to define the transport category. In this way the selection positions were reduced, accelerating the selection process.

The requirement for a new prototype was the placement of the lighting indication around the housing and on the top of the housing. The new design can be seen in figure 5.17. The led driver circuit was also improved; the TLC59711 led driver from TI was discarded, and a six PWM channels performed the LED regulation, figure 5.16(b) depicts the new circuit. Also, the brightness of LEDs from the first prototype, CREE CLV1AFKB, was compared to other LEDs using the new driver system. The selected LEDs were from AVAGO part number: ASMT-YTB7-0AA02.

5.4 Summary

The systematic implementation of the new wearable platform is explained. Three prototypes are presented, with the first, a tabletop prototype the basic software functions were implemented and tested, they included the parsing of sensor and GPS data, its analysis and the radio communication. The pre-triage algorithm was validated on the microcontroller with simulated and real data. Different technical characteristic, as the power consumption are as well presented. After laboratory tests a first wearable version was integrated, ten tags were produced and tested at MCI scenarios. Based on results a second wearable prototype was implemented.

For the evaluation of the optimized wearable tag, twenty units were produced and tested together with ten tags of the first version. Evaluations occurred during MCI simulations, where the hard conditions of a real scenario were recreated. During these simulated scenarios, communication, localization and sensor data were tested. The general purpose was to test the feasibility of such systems to operate during MCI scenarios and to accomplish its task to provide medical and tactical information to support commanders, physicians and paramedics to perform their tasks. The next chapter discusses in detail the test scenarios and the obtained results.

6 System Evaluation

Last chapter depicted the implementation of the wearable triage tag; many questions about its performance and operations feasibility during MCI scenarios aroused. This chapter presents the different performed evaluations and results concerning the validation of the new platform from different aspects. As mentioned before, the hypothesis to test is whether, with such a system, it is possible to provide commanders, physicians, and paramedics with accurate medical and tactical information. The main goal is to support the rescue planning and the medical care on site. In order to accept or reject the hypothesis, it is required to approach the system's test from different levels and aspects. The platform evaluation required the test of different system's features from a technical and usability perspective. Some of the different aspects to evaluate are:

- Technical aspects:
  - Communication Performance
  - Performance of the localization modules
  - Performance of the sensor modules
- Usability aspects:
  - Accuracy of the Pre-Triage Information
  - Performance during rough use
  - End-user acceptance

In the last chapter, some technical aspects were tested in laboratory conditions. In order to see the real performance of the new wearable triage tag, it is necessary to recreate conditions from real MCI scenarios. In this chapter, different test scenarios and methods are presented. They include MCI simulations, where real emergency commanders, physicians and paramedics used the wearable tag as a triage tool. Another test scenarios were real emergencies. Here, paramedics collected sensor data and references from real victims. This information supported the evaluation of the pre-triage algorithm with data from real emergency patients.

6.1 Field Evaluation - MCI Simulations

6.1.1 Evaluation Methodology

In order to validate the usability, user acceptance and performance of the communication and sensor modules of the new device in real conditions, different MCI scenarios were recreated. The company Antworting organized the MCI simulations; this company is an expert in rescue logistics. Different types of MCI scenarios were simulated, including traffic accidents, fire in buildings and industrial accidents. At the simulations, tenths of actors played the role of victims, and hundreds of rescue personals performed normal rescue procedures during the scenario.

The wearable triage tag was integrated as part of a rescue platform including a web portal service and a handheld device for the physicians and commanders in the field. Figure 4.3 depicts the concept of the MCI information and communication system; figure 6.1 presents the developed system.

The simulations sequence were designed to test the features and performance of the first realization of the wearable tag. In this way, the experience could be collected to design and improve the wearable device into a second prototype. Last chapter, specifically in sections 5.3.2 and 5.3.3, explained the conception and integration of both prototype version.

The first prototype was tested in two different simulation events. The first took place at Warendorf were three MCI scenarios were organized; one at the DRK building; another, a fire incident at a grill party; and the last one, a traffic accident. At each scenario, ten victims were simulated with different injured levels, and around one hundred rescuers attended the scenarios, going from paramedics and firemen. The objective of the scenarios was to gain a first experience with the prototype in terms of communication, triage and localization information and usability.

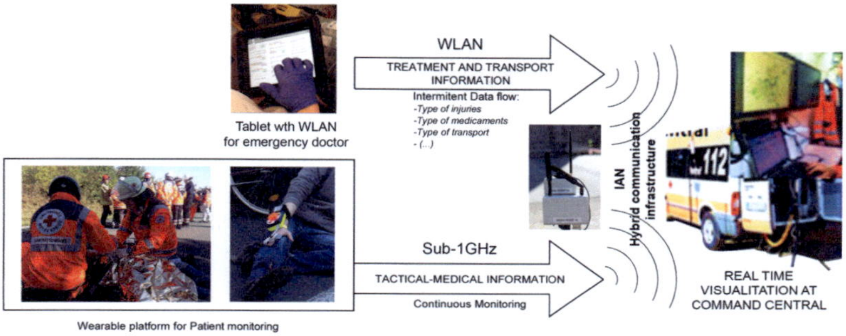

Figure 6.1: Developed IAN for MCI with wearable platform for continuous monitoring of patients

After the first evaluation, only a few changes at the software level were performed. In order to gain more experience in the usability with different user's perspective, a second simulation event took place at Coesfeld. Here, four scenarios were organized, the first one was a traffic accident, the second was a fire in a residence house and the third was a chemical accident in an industrial area. Around 300 rescuers participated at this event.

Based on the evaluation results of the first two evaluation events, an improved wearable triage tag was integrated. Section 5.3.3 presented the improvements and a new prototype design. A third evaluation event was organized at Oelde. There, both prototypes were tested, and similar to the first events, different MCI scenarios were organized. The first simulation was an emergency at an open air theater; the second was a building in a fire, the third a traffic accident and the last a resident house in a fire accident.

Figure 6.2 to 6.4 provide some pictures of the MCI simulations. It is possible to appreciate how rescuers used both wearable systems as triage tools. In the first and second events, ten units of the first prototype were tested while, in the last event, ten units of the first version plus twenty units of the second prototype were included. For testing purposes, data was recorded in the SD card included on the tag, and at the server side.

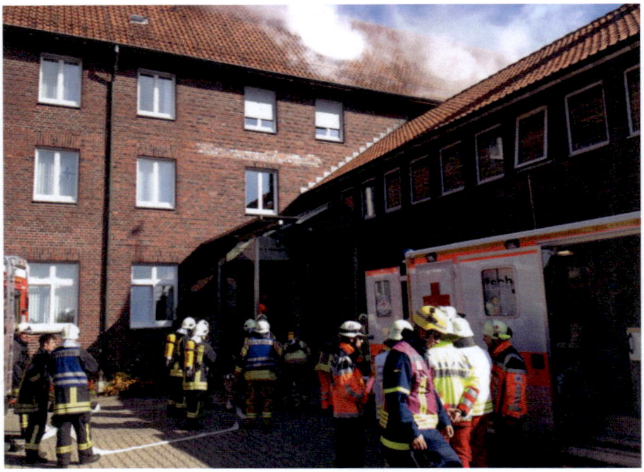

(a) Recreated fire incident at elderly residence

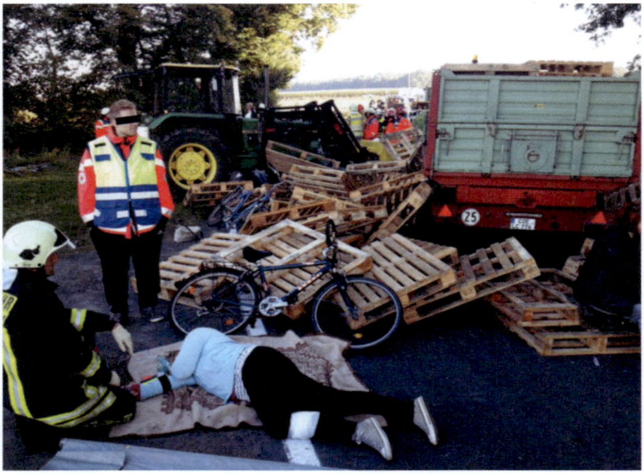

(b) Recreation of traffic accident

Figure 6.2: Wearable Prototype tested at recreated MCI [HRR+14]

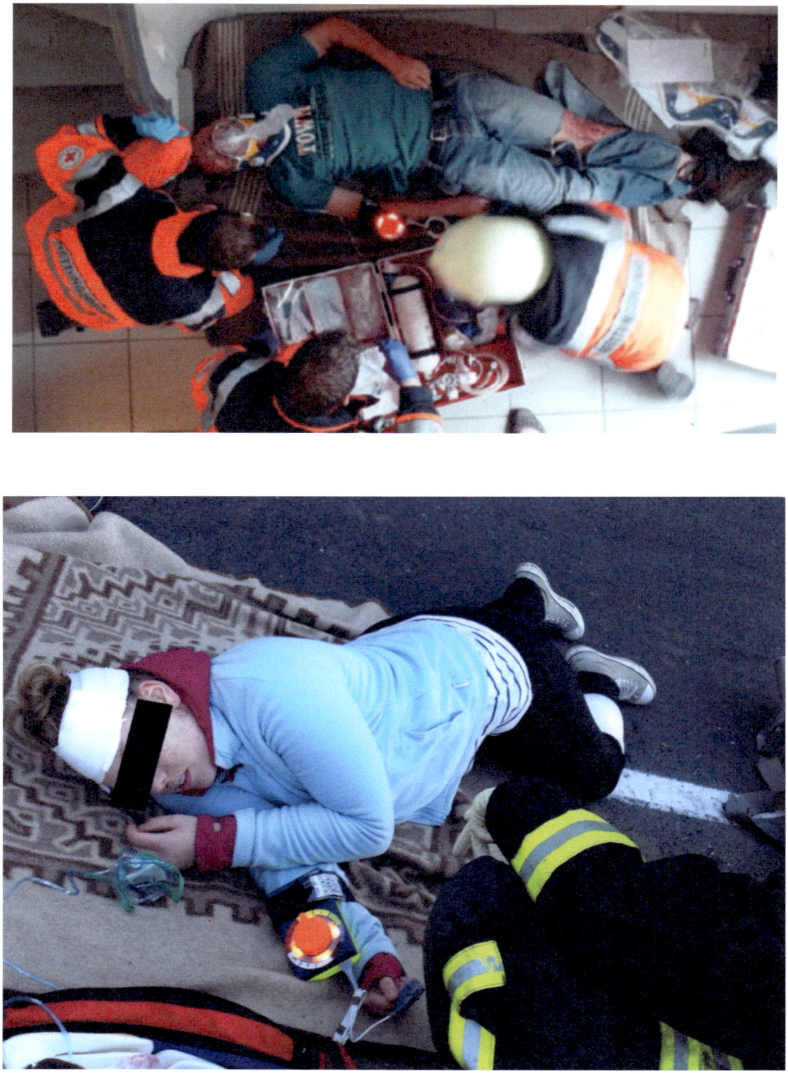

Figure 6.3: First Wearable Prototype tested at recreated MCI [HRR+14]

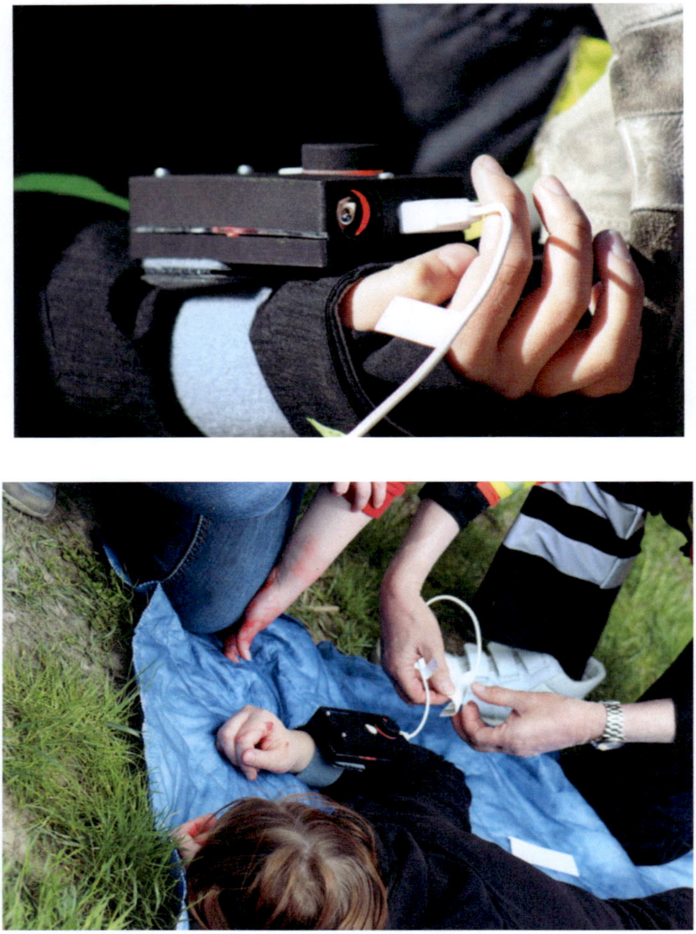

Figure 6.4: Optimized Wearable Prototype tested at recreated MCI

During the simulation, data was recorded, and health personnel were interviewed about the system performance. Results on differently evaluated aspects, as sensor measurement, localization, algorithms, RF communication and usability are discussed next.

6.1.2 Real-time Communication, System Usability and User Acceptance

Based on the feedback of end-users and the discussions with experts during the evaluations, it was concluded that the main advantages are the real-time communication, the ergonomics of the wearable tag and the robustness of the system.

Real-time Information

The real-time communication of the triage and pre-triage information was a main benefice according to the emergency personnel. The fusion of data coming from all tags automatically provides a vision of the number of critical patients and a vision of the corresponding triage categories. The localization of the patients also allows to identify how many of them are still in the incident zone, in the triage, or the treatment or transport area. The automatic patient identification also permitted to make reference to the correct patient.

This benefit was reflected in the perception of a clear reduction of the voice communication. Walkie-talkies were used to manage more specific situations; therefore, communication traffic is reduced.

The robustness of the real-time communication was tested for both prototypes. The packet loss rate was estimated comparing the expected number of packets and the received packets at the server side, the results show a mean approx. of 1% packet loss for the first prototype and less than 0.5% for the second triage tag.

Wearable Triage Tag Ergonomics

The application and use of the wearable triage tag were also under observation. During the first evaluations events, feedback about the first prototype was provided by interviews with the paramedics:

- rotatory switch is easy to operate
- tag can be attached to patient quickly
- size reduction is necessary

- neutral colors for the housing: white, black or gray
- only selected triage label must be visible
- rotary switch for triage level and a slide switch for transport category
- armband flexible for different body size
- led indication must be around the housing but also visible from the top

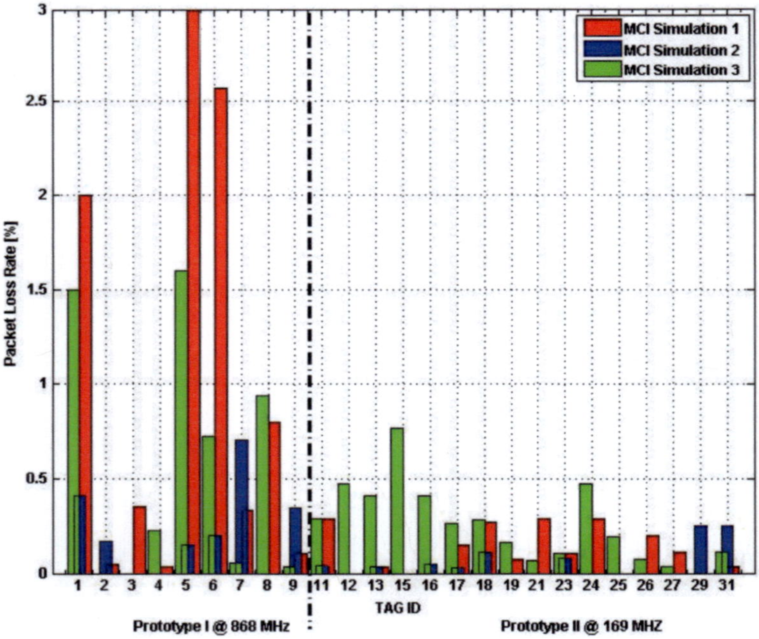

Figure 6.5: Packet loss rate for both wearable prototypes

Based on this feedback, the second prototype was designed and integrated, see section 5.3.2. In comparison to the actual triage tag, the new tag represents an advantage in the ergonomics; it is easier and quicker to use. For example, to set the triage or transport category, it is only required to turn on the switch. While in the paper tag, it is necessary to take out a card from the plastic bag, and then select the right category and introduce the card again. This process consumes time and challenges the paramedics, which are under stress conditions during MCI scenarios. Another example is the attachment system, as mentioned in section 3.1.2, where the cord of today's triage tag might be tangled, and to untangle it might be an impossible task under MCI scenarios conditions. The armband of the new prototype solves this problem.

Robustness against Rough Conditions

The robustness of the device was also under test. Following this purpose, the physical state of all tags was examined after each simulation. All tags were fully operable after each MCI exercise, and a not significant damage was observed. Additionally, non-battery failure existed, proving that the fixing system and the electronics resisted rough conditions.

The first prototype was operated around twelve hours of MCI simulations and the second prototype during four hours. Health personnel were asked to treat the device as they would do it normally. To the robustness results, the performance of the RF communication modules can be added, which achieved a packet loss rate lower than 0.5% with no significant latency. ZigBee technologies for the same purposes have shown latencies even of ten minutes [RHKW11].

6.1.3 Sensor Modules Performance

During the MCI simulations, the performance of the sensor modules was also tested. Pulse oximeter and acceleration sensor were tested independently because in these simulations; actors play only the role of victims; their physiological signals were healthy and do not correlated to the situation they characterized. The only parameter that might be correlated with the situation was the activity.

However, the test conditions were suitable to test the measurement quality of the pulse oximeter and to test the activity parameter to identify critical and non-critical victims. For testing purposes, all sensor data and pre-triage results were stored in the SD card. The GPS clock was the reference to synchronized the sensor data. Details and results are explained next.

Pulse Oximeter Measurement Feasibility and Robustness

The pulse oximeter provides a quality index for each SpO2 and heart rate values, see Table 5.2. The quality index was stored for each measurement. As a reference of the robustness of the module under MCI conditions, the quality index was analyzed for different wearable tags. Figure 6.6 presents 30 minutes of recorded data during a simulated MCI. It is possible to see the relation between the quality index, the perfusion index, the measured HR and SpO2 and the acceleration. From minute 22 it is possible to appreciate the effect of the movement in the data from the pulse oximeter, the measurement is lost and the quality is low and the PI is low. It can be concluded that the PI and QI can support the detection of artifacts in the measurement and prevent the algorithm from possible failures.

Figure 6.7 represents the same effect. Plots at the left show a clean pleth cure, which was measured even during periods with moderated movements. On the right, the first plot shows a pleth curved with movement artifacts. In the second plot, the PI presents another behavior as the expected, it is increases with the movement. Only the quality index follows the expected behavior: low during movement and medium along periods moderated movement.

Figure 6.8 presents the analysis of pulse oximeter recorded data during 3 recreated exercises that lasted at least 40 minutes. The figure shows that approximately 60% of the wearable platforms had more than 60% of valid data. The figure also shows that platforms with more valid data also presented higher PI and quality. It means that most of the tags recorded at least 24 minutes of data. For the periods without pulse oximeter data, the accelerometer supports the pre-triage algorithm. Constant movement artifacts would be an indication the movement capacity of the patient.

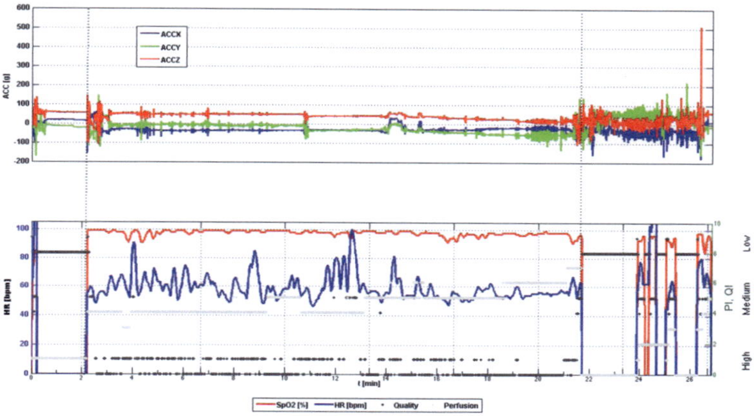

Figure 6.6: Quality of sensors measurements and its dependency to movement artifacts

Activity Class and Triage Category and its dependency to movement artifacts

As mentioned, the pre-triage class based on the activity classification was also stored in the SD card. In order to test the activity classifier as an indicator of the gravity of the victim, a hypothesis was defined. The hypothesis stated that the patients manually classified with the green category, or non-severe injured patients would frequently move and be automatically classified as non-critical patients. On the contrary, red classified patients might not move and will be classified as critical.

In figure 6.9 the results for non-severe injured victims are presented. The position of the triage turn-switch and the automatic pre-triage were saved on the SD card, as a function of the activity classification. The figure 6.9 shows that paramedics classified the patient with the triage category III (green). However, the pre-triage class results showed that the majority classification are critical, contrary to the expected result. It was observed that the patient moved around at the beginning of the exercise, before being attended or triage by a paramedic. When they were under medical supervision in the treatment area, they did not move a lot.

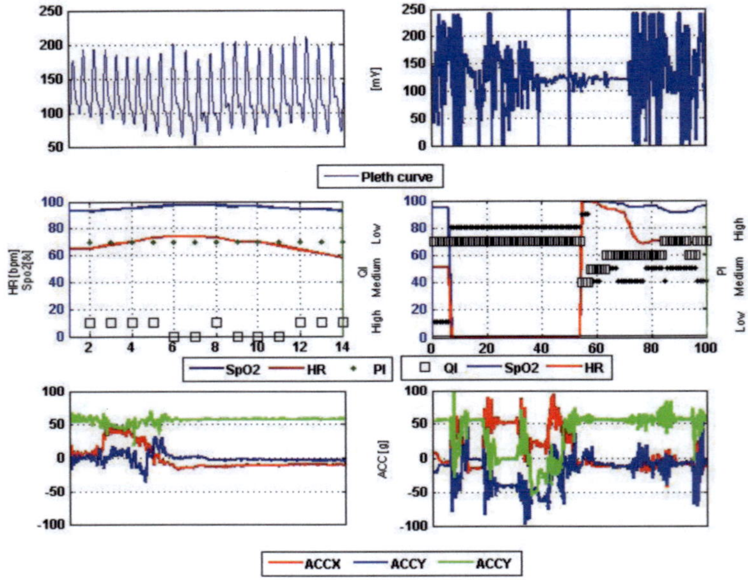

Figure 6.7: Quality of the pleth signal

Table 6.1 shows the results from comparing triage and pre-triage for severe and non-severe injured patients. These results confirm that the pre-triage algorithm is suitable to indicate the criticality of the patient. Patients with triage category I were classified 96% of the time as critical, whereas patients with category III were only 29% of the time, correctly classified. For the same patients, the same comparison was done taking out the movement- classification dependency. Results showed that when considering only the SpO2 and HR, the accuracy of the classification increased to 95%. Automatic pre-triage classification of non-critical ones might require another processing strategy for a movement-based classification.

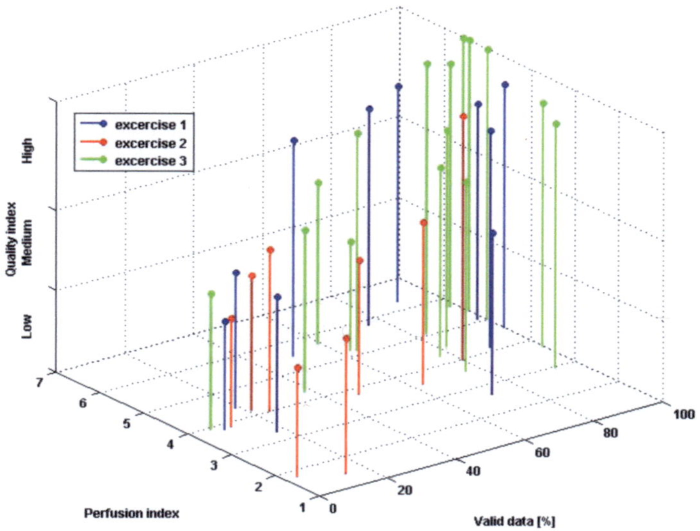

Figure 6.8: Valid measurement rate Vs. perfusion index

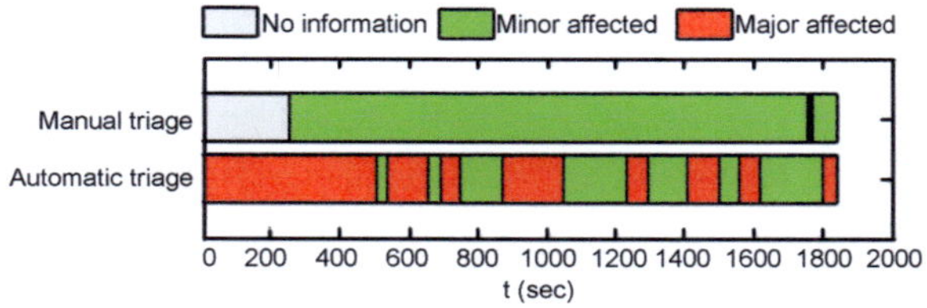

Figure 6.9: Automatic pre-triage as a function of activity classification Vs. triage

For the second simulation exercise, the pre-triage based on the activity classification was only active until the first triage input. After the first medical supervision the activity classification was inactive and the pre-triage was based only on the HR and SpO2 values. It was observed with the same analysis that the results reflected more accurately the expected pre-triage classification for a non- severely injured patient; the patient with category III was 89% of the time correctly classified.

Table 6.1: Automatic pre-triage as a function of the movement classification

manual triage category:	CAT I	CAT III		
automatic pre-triage	movement-based	movement-based	SpO2 & HR but no movement-based	movement-based only before first manual triage
non-critical	4 %	29 %	95 %	89 %
critical	96 %	61 %	5 %	11 %

The results indicates that it must be taken into account, if the classification is after or before a manual triage. In other words, before the first manual triage or after a long period without medical supervision, the activity classifier must be considered in the pre-triage algorithm to evaluate the criticality of the patient.

6.1.4 Patient Localization

The different simulated scenarios gave the opportunity to the test the GPS system for the localization of the patients. The scenarios that implied patients inside a house or building were of major interest. A method to test the localization is the multiplication of the DOP factor and the accuracy of the device. As mentioned before, the DOP is an indication of the precision of the localization error *LOCerror*. Based on the formula 6.1, GPS data from the wearable device was analyzed and shown in table 6.2.

$$LOCerror = DOP \times \text{accuracy gps module} \tag{6.1}$$

Figure 6.10 shows that even in indoor scenarios, the tag was able to indicate that the patients were inside the building, with an accuracy of eleven meters. For outdoor scenarios, the localization accuracy was about 3.0 m, which fulfills the requirements described in 4.2. Figure 6.10(b) shows that the localization module could differentiate between patients who are still at the incident are and those who are already in the treatment area.

Table 6.2: GPS localization performance

Device ID	Tag 1	Tag 2	Tag 3
Time to first fix	64 s	35 s	42 s
	MCI excercise 1		
Average DOP	1.45	1.43	1.33
Average error	3.625 m	3.575 m	3.325 m
	MCI excercise 2		
Average DOP	1.63	1.38	1.42
Average error	4.08 m	3.45 m	3.55 m
	MCI excercise 3		
Average DOP	1.4	0.88	0.94
Average error	3.5 m	2.2 m	2.35 m
	Average		
Average DOP	1.31		
Average error	3.295 m		

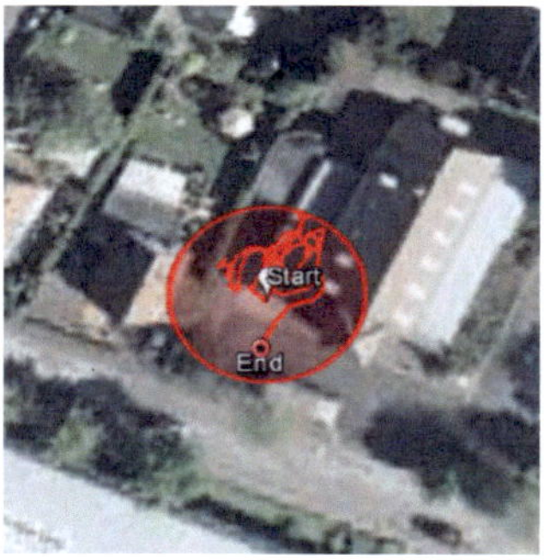

(a) Localization near building area

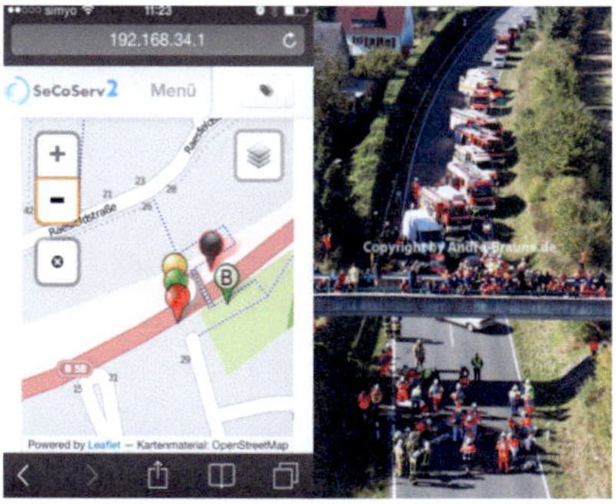

(b) Localization during MCI, the bridge separates the triage and the treatment area areas

Figure 6.10: Examples of localization performance

6.2 Pre-Triage Algorithm Validation

Emergency drills do not provide a real reference for the evaluation of the automatic pre-triage algorithm. Healthy actors play the role of victims, and even if they are affected by the stress of the drill, variations on their vital signs do not correlate with the represented role. Due to the spontaneity nature of real MCI scenarios it is not possible to plan the collection of vital signs under real conditions.

However, patient data must not necessarily be taken from real MCI scenarios, but from emergency scenarios. It does not matter if they are a single casualty incident; they would provide a reference to test the algorithm with data from an emergency situation. For this purpose, data collection from emergency situations was planned in cooperation with the company Antworting and the relief agency Malteser, based at the city of Vechta, in North Germany. Along four months, they performed this task, and a valid dataset of ninety real casualties was gathered. SpO2, heart rate, and acceleration data were recorded, and triage references were provided. Specific time references for the arrival to the emergency site and departure to hospitals were digitally annotated as well. The following subsections explains into details the study to validate the pre-triage algorithm.

6.2.1 Study Design and Evaluation Method

The objective of this study was to specify the capability of the pre-triage algorithm to identify the critical and non-critical patients. The capability must be presented in terms of accuracy, specificity and sensitivity. Aside the global accuracy, the performance of each parameter, SpO2, HR, and activity were evaluated. In this way, it was possible to determine which parameter was more suitable for the patient classification.

In order to perform the evaluation, reference annotations with which to compare the pre-triage results are necessary. It was defined together with the Malteser's personnel to collect two annotations type: first impression triage and the NACA-score. Both are explained next:

- First impression triage: this annotation parameter relies only on the experience of the paramedic. Rescue personnel must annotate it after a rough examination of the patient and the situation. It is a general first estimation of the patient condition. In this way, it is possible to evaluate the pre-triage algorithm with the paramedic's experience.

- NACA-Score: it is a standard protocol to determine the criticality of the emergency patient. It is based on a standard examination of different conditions and vital parameters, similar to the START algorithm, which was depicted in section 2.1.2. Table 6.3 shows the different stadiums of the NACA-Score. For the simplification of the comparison with the pre-triage classes, all patients between score I-III were considered to be annotated as non-critical and scores IV-V as critical.

Table 6.3: Definition NACA categories

Category	Description
NACA I	*insignificant disruption*
NACA II	*ambulant care, transport to hospital is not required*
NACA III	*moderate disruptions, stationary treatment is required* *non emergency measures are required*
NACA IV	*serious disruption, acute danger is not discarded,* *emergency measures are required*
NACA V	*acute danger*

Algorithm Evaluation

The algorithm is evaluated based on the calculation of the accuracy, sensitivity *Se* and specificity *Sp*. These metrics can be calculated from a confusion matrix in which all recognized and unrecognized events are registered, see table 6.4.

Based on the automatic pre-triage algorithm, sensitivity *Se* set a reference for the quality detection of critical patients that, from the perspective of paramedics, are critical. The correct identification of the critical patients is especially relevant since an underestimation of the criticality of the patient condition would also suppose an underestimation of emergency and the necessary resources, compromising the health care provision. On the other hand, non-critical patients incorrectly identified would suppose an overestimation of the emergency situation, but do not compromise the logistics of the rescue operation. Specificity is a reference for the performance of correct detected non-critical patients that, from the perspective of the annotations of the paramedics, are non-critical.

Table 6.4: True table

	Predicted Class	No Predicted Class
Expected Class	True Positive (TP)	False Positive (FP)
	False Negative (FN)	True Negative (TN)

In order to determine the *Se* and *Sp*, sensor data and reference must be parsed and synchronized. All matches and deviations are counted according to the confusion matrix and are calculated as follows:

$$\text{Se} = \frac{TP}{TP + FN} \tag{6.2}$$

$$\text{Sp} = \frac{TN}{FP + TN} \tag{6.3}$$

$$\text{Accuracy} = \frac{TP + TN}{TP + TN + FP + FN} \tag{6.4}$$

Where TP (true positive) is the number of all critical patients detected correctly. FN (false negative) is the number all non-critical patients that are not recognized as non-critical, and FP (false positive) is the number of critical patients non-correctly detected. TN (true negative) stands for the non-critical patients that are correctly classified, according to the paramedic's annotation perspective.

6.2.2 Data Collection

In order to collect the patient's data, a commercial sensor platform was selected. The paramedics carried them in the two ambulances during the study. In this way, each time they had an emergency, they were able to attach the sensors to the wrist of the patient, in the same way as the wearable triage tag. Once the device was attached to the victim, it started to stored SpO2 and HR with a rate of 1 Hz and acceleration data with a rate of 64 Hz. Paramedics also carried a handheld device, where they recorded the required annotations: first impression triage only based on a general and intuitive impression from the moment they meet the scene, and the NACA score, which is an assessment protocol.

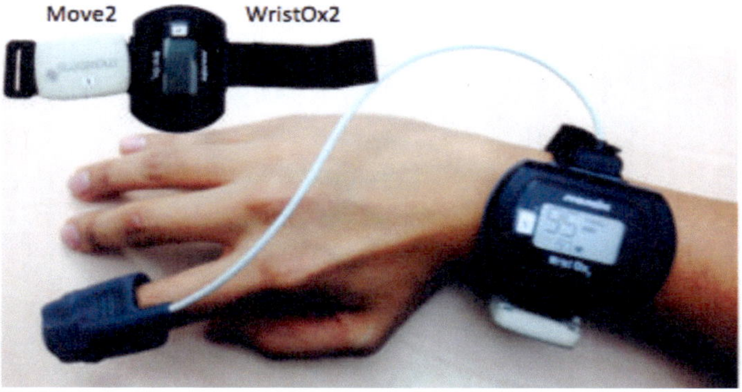

Figure 6.11: Sensor data collection platform for pre-triage study

The sensor platform consisted of a WristOX2 Nonin pulse oximeter and a Move2 Movisens activity analyzer, see figure 6.11. After each shift, paramedics had to connect both sensors to a terminal computer that stored the sensor data at cloud storage services automatically. In this way, sensor data could be automatically downloaded at the laboratory for its analysis. Figure 6.12 depicts the data collection and data flow.

Paramedics regularly updated reference annotations. They were recorded in an Excel table containing the patient id, date and time of service (arrival on the scene, departure to hospital and arrival to the hospital), and both annotations. Date and time information was the reference to synchronize the annotations with the sensors data.

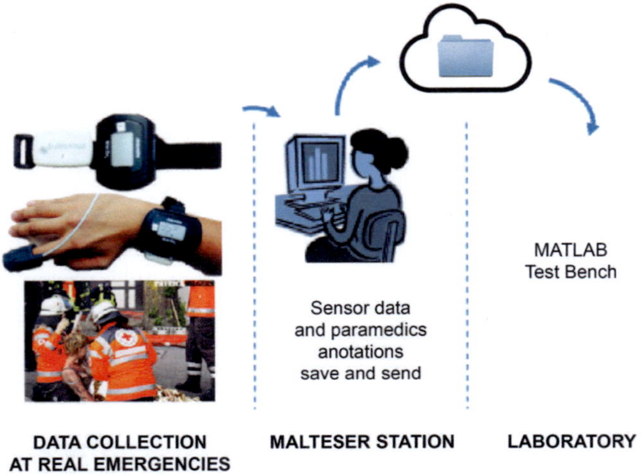

(a) Data collection process

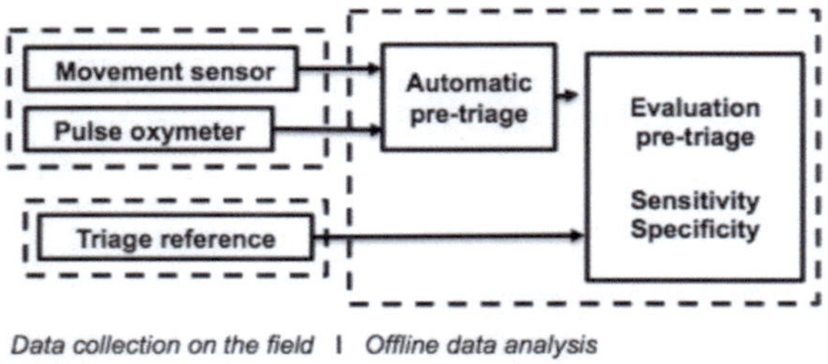

(b) Signal flow for analysis of automatic pre-triage vs. manual triage reference

Figure 6.12: Data collection during real emergencies and flow for data analysis

Two ambulances took part during the development of the study development; the relief agency Malteser in Vechta performed the data collection between the 1.01.2014 and the 18.03.2014. As a result, a total of 190 patients were recorded.

6.2.3 Data Analysis and Evaluation

Annotations from paramedics and sensor collected data was analyzed offline at the laboratory. A test bench was implemented in Matlab for the parsing, synchronization and evaluation of the data. It was observed that many sensor data was corrupted so only sensor data with at least two minutes of continuity was considered as valid. After this constraint, the dataset was reduced to 90 patients.

Since sensor data came from two different platforms (pulse oximeter and activity sensor), they must be synchronized first. The unisens data format, which is suitable for the synchronization of sensor data from different platforms, was used. The clock of the pulse oximeter is taken as a reference for the synchronization. Later, the data was packed together and again synchronized, but this time with the annotations table. Time stamps from the paramedic's table are computer's clock based. The pre-triage algorithm for the sensor data was calculated in the same way, as in the wearable triage tag; a classification result was calculated with a rate of 2 Hz. After synchronization, different evaluations were performed, they are explained in the next section.

Evaluation Results - Overall Accuracy

Sensor data was analyzed and classified every thirty seconds. For the estimation of the accuracy, each classification result was compared with the references of the paramedics. Global analysis and partial analysis were performed. The global analysis comprises the accuracy of the complete automatic pre-triage algorithm. Also, each parameter was analyzed separately to test their influence on the algorithm. Becuase the patients are normally under observation, and a considerable movement was not expected, and it was expected that the activity parameter would not be accurate.

From the 90 observed patients only for 58 patients, activity sensor information was available. Annotations presented some differences between the first impression triage and the NACA Score. First triage impression annotated 36 patients as critical and 54 as non-critical, while for the NACA score 47 patients were critical and 43 non-critical. That gives the impression that paramedics do not identify easily critical patients and that they need to follow a standard protocol to detect critical patients. This difference between annotations might be an indicator that paramedics underestimate the emergency of the attended patients.

Table 6.5 shows the obtained results from the comparison between the sensor data and the annotations. In general the accuracy of the first triage is higher than the NACA score. It is important to remark that the first triage is only the first intuition of the paramedic about the emergency of the patient. In the other hand, the NACA score is a deep inspection of the patient, paramedics annotate it at the end of the operation. The difference might be an indication of the recovery or stabilization of the patient during the attention of the paramedics.

Table 6.5: Overall classification accuracy

	Accuracy [%]				
	all	**SpO2 & HR**	**SpO2**	**HR**	**Movement**
First Triage	64.9	69.9	69.6	82.9	63.6
NACA Score	62.6	58.4	62.5	82.7	53.2

The HR is the parameter providing the highest accuracy, followed by the combination of the SpO2 and HR. In order to test deeper the accuracy for each patient, the figure presents the histogram resulting from the accuracy per patient and test. It is observable that for the case of the first impression triage, the SpO2, HR and their combination have more patients with an accuracy over 70%. For the case of the NACA score, only the HR is clearly accurate. The histograms in figure 6.13 support the results from table 6.5, showing that the individual analysis of SpO2 and HR classifies a greater amount of patient with an accuracy higher than 80%. The HR has the highest number of patients classified with an accuracy higher than 90 %

Evaluation Results - Sensitivity and Specificity

Another test was performed setting a label for each patient based on the sensor data. The label defined the critical status of the patient only if at least 20% of the automatic pre-triage results indicate a critical status;

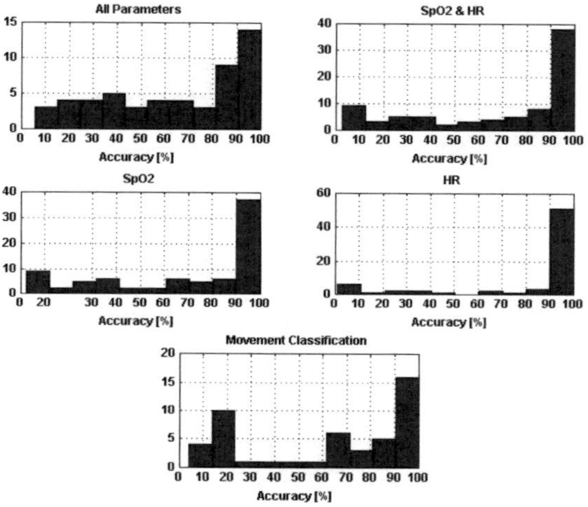

(a) First impression triage histograms - accuracy per patient

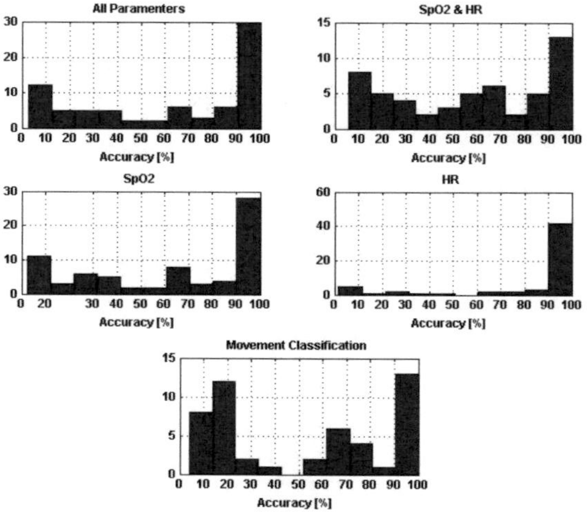

(b) Naca score histograms - accuracy per patient

Figure 6.13: Accuracy histogram for first impression triage and NACA score otherwise the patient is considered non-critical. Then the label of each patient was compared with the annotations of paramedics. In this way, it was possible to determine the specificity, sensitivity and the accuracy of the new automatic pre-triage algorithm.

For the rescue planning, the sensitivity is more relevant since it indicates the probability to distinguish the critical patients correctly. Low values would produce an underestimation of the emergency. In the case of the specificity, wrong detection would cause an overestimation of the criticality of the patients at an MCI scenario.

It is to remember that the paramedics annotate the first impression triage at the beginning of the service, only after a general inspection of the casualty and the scenario. The NACA score is the result of a more specific inspection performed along the emergency service and annotated at the end of the service.

The sensitivity and specificity were investigated for each parameter. The sensitivity describes the rate of true positives and the specificity of true negatives. Severely affected patients were defined as a positive result of the classification and the minor affected as a negative result. Table 6.6 presents the obtained results.

The SpO2 was the most relevant parameter to identify critical patients. However, the HR and the activity are necessary to increase the global sensitivity. In the case of the specificity, the parameter the better supports the classification of non-critical was the HR. However, the global specificity is aligned by the parameter with the lowest value, this because all parameters have to be non-critical to define the patient as non-major affected.

Table 6.6: Sensitivity and specificity of the sensor-based triage taking as reference the NACA score provided by paramedics

	Global	**Partial**		
	all [%]	**SpO2 [%]**	**HR [%]**	**Activity [%]**
sensitivity [%]	61.3	**58.4**	20.2	27.7
specificity [%]	74.4	74.4	**90.2**	79.7

Aside the NACA score paramedics annotated at the arrival to the site a first evaluation of the emergency. This first evaluation was denominated as first impression triage, consisting of a subjective evaluation of the status of the patient. This observation was only based on the experience of the paramedic. Paramedics classified the patient as critical or non-critical. This first impression triage is similar to the evaluation that they normally provide at the very beginning of a rescue operation. Where, they pursuit to establish if the scenario is critical or non-critical depending on the quantity of severe injured or ill patients.

Based on this first impression triage, the sensor-based triage was tested. The automatic triage provides a general estimation of the patient status from the beginning of the rescue. The sensor-based triage was compared with the first impression triage to calculated the sensitivity and specificity, in the same way as with the NACA score. Table 6.7 shows the obtained results.

Table 6.7: Sensitivity and specificity of the sensor-based triage taking as reference the first impression triage provided by paramedics

	Global		**Partial**	
	all [%]	**SpO2 [%]**	**HR [%]**	**Activity [%]**
sensitivity [%]	72.1	**65.5**	33.2	30.1
specificity [%]	77.5	77.5	**93.0**	81.5

Results show the same tendency as in the obtained results with the NACA score. SpO2 accounts clearly for the identification of the critical patients and the HR for the non-critical ones. SpO2 also established the specificity of the sensor-based triage. The results are higher comparing the sensor-based triage with the first impression triage of the paramedics.

The presented results would support the implementation of a compensation system to overcome the observed underestimation of the critical patients. If an MCI has 100 critical casualties, a pre-triage based only on the HR would estimate 70 patients with a critical situation, an addition of 30 casualties would overcome the underestimations. This is only possible if the number of patients and the *Se* are known.

6.3 Summary

The evaluation methods and tools are explained. Two test scenarios are explained: recreated MCI and real individual emergencies. Technical feasibility and user acceptance were under test at simulated MCI. Results show a general well function and user acceptance. The wearable showed robust performance even the hard conditions of the MCI scenarios.

Validation of pre-triage algorithm followed in cooperation with Malteser and DRK. SpO2, HR and activity data from 90 patients was collected and compares with paramedics references. An *Se* of 72.5% and an *Sp* of 77.5% showed the potential of the new system to provide an acceptable triage of the emergency scenario.

7 Conclusion & Outlook

First response during MCI and disaster scenarios represent an enormous challenge for the rescue services. Operation management requires a fast and accurate estimation of the urgency of the situation. Distribution of medical care and transport to the hospitals is the main concern of the incident command. Only with the description and diagnose of the casualties, it is possible to proceed with the rescue activities. Thus, information and communication system is necessary for the documentation of the patient's status. Paramedics and emergency doctors have a responsibility to generate, collect and communicate the patient information. Operational command and a senior emergency doctor are responsible for the rescue management; they gather the patient information and follow with the rescue plan.

Ordinary tools, as walkie-talkies, paper triage cards, paper protocols and whiteboards are commonly used as documentation and communication platform. Lessons learned and different study has been showing that these tools do not fulfill the information and communication demand, overwhelming the rescue forces and generating uncertainty.

Different research projects have shown that the introduction of modern information and communication tools represents a solution to accelerate the data collection and automatic visualization of relevant information. Tablets and PDAs and ad hoc wireless networks facilitate the interaction between the personnel on the field and the command center. Among the research projects, some have used RFID tags to identify the patients, but others have gone beyond and implemented active triage tags to substitute the actual paper triage cards.

Active triage tags have been integrated with different physiological sensors. They transmit in real time raw data to the command central. Some of them would indicate the triage condition automatically. However, neither the transmission of physiological raw data is desired nor the automatic triage. The first is time-consuming and requires a considerable effort to abstract manually relevant data. The second requires the constant verification and confirmation of the automatic alerts.

Discussions with experts from the emergency field indicated that rescuers welcome the new technologies. However, researchers have not taken full advantage of them. For example in the case of triage cards with RFID tags, there is a lack of constant monitoring, compromising with the time the validity of the data that paramedics collected with PDAs. In other words, the intermittent data collection does not support the detection of rapid patient deterioration. The detection can only occur if the doctors are constantly monitoring and triaging each casualty. This scenario is not possible because at MCI normally paramedics are outnumbered by the amount of casualties. In the case of the active monitoring, developed active triage overwhelm the rescue personnel with an excess of physiological raw data or with alerts that need a constant verification.

This dissertation presented a new wearable platform for the remote monitoring of casualties. It integrates as well physiological sensors, to perform a constant monitoring of the patient status. In contrast to other active triage technologies, the new platform performs an automatic analysis of the physiological data and provides a sense-making result that would support the tactical planning from the beginning of the rescue operation. Beside the classification algorithm, its design must fulfill the requirements of the end-users. It must be robust and operable under the hard conditions present at MCI scenarios.

The new platform design is the result of the discussion with many experts from the emergency field. As well, the definition of the new algorithm is a result of these discussions. The new algorithm, denominated as the automatic pre-triage algorithm, informs the command center every thirty seconds about the condition of the patient. A pulse oximeter and activity classifier based on an accelerometer support the classification of the patient. The algorithm decides if the patient is critical or non-critical. The objective of this classification is to abstract medical-tactical information. This information has the purpose to support the commander from the first moment of the operation to estimate the urgency of the scenario and to facilitate the estimation of resources necessary to provide effective health care to the casualties.

Beside the automatic patient classification, the new platform must allow the manual triage and provide visual information of the triage category and the transport priority; this information would support the normal rescue process. In contrast, the automatic pre-triage is only visible at the command central and would not generate conflict with the ordinary triage classification.

Many technical questions around the feasibility of the monitoring of physiological conditions, the localization and the communication were answered recreating MCI scenarios. For the validation of the automatic pre-triage algorithm, it was necessary to collect physiological data from real casualties. This dissertation also presents the results of the study performed together with relief agency Malteser. A long four months they collected data from one hundred ninety real casualties.

Results from recreated MCI scenarios showed an acceptable performance of the radio communication, the physiological sensing and the localization. At the scenarios, less than the 10% of the packets were lost. The localization error was about 3 m, and most of the sensor data was valid, even the hard conditions of the recreated scenarios. At these scenarios, it was possible to observe the potential that the activity classification had to indicate the status of the patient. It was concluded that if the patient has not been yet diagnosed, the classification of its activity will be a good reference for its criticality.

In general rescue personnel welcome the new platform and indicated an acceleration of the documentation process, reflected in a reduction of the voice traffic communication. As well, two municipalities are interested in pilot projects involving the production of one thousand wearable platforms for each one. The production of end-product based on the actual design would require a hardware review and a scalability test that involves more than fifty nodes. Until now only thirty have been tested together.

The validation of the automatic pre-triage algorithm with data from real casualties showed the importance of the considreation of SpO2, HR and patient activity for the classification of critical and non-critical casualties. Classification results showed that the system would recognized 72.5% of the severly injured casualties. The actual description of the accuracy of the system to detect critical patients would led to compensate any understimation on site.

However, the future investigation must consider a second validation of the algorithm. An increment of the annotation of references is necessary, only in this way it would be possible to study the accuracy of the algorithm to detect transitions from critical to non-critical and vice versa. This kind study would provide a more accurate knowledge of the impact of the algorithm to classify emergency patients.

It is difficult to test the usability of the information generated by the pre-triage algorithm. MCI scenarios are unexpected, and it is not possible to plan their study. Thus, special software applications to simulate the algorithm output must be developed and tested with end-users, permitting to evaluate the effect of the pre-triage information in their decision-making process.

Figures

Tables

Abbreviations

ACTS	Advanced Communications Technology Satellite
AID-N	Advanced Health and Disaster Aid Network
AIO	Ambulance Incident Officer
ALS	Advanced Life Support
ARTEMIS	Automated Triage and Emergency Management Information System
ATM	Asynchronous Transfer Mode
ATS	Application Satellite Technology
AWSN	Autonomous Wireless Sensor Network
BAN	Body Area Networks
BGAN	Broadband Global Area Network
BLS	Basic Life Support
BMBF	Federal Ministry of Education and Reasearch
BP	Blood Pressure
COMSAT	Communications Satellite
CTS	Communication Technology Satellite
DIN	German Institute for Standardization
DRK	German Red Cross
DVB-RCS	Digital Video Broadcasting - Return Channel Satellite
e-Triage	Electronic Affected Detection in Catastrophes
EC	Emergency Commander
ECG	Electrocardiogram
GEO	Geostationary
GPS	Global Positionig System
GSM	Global System for Mobile Communications
GTE	General Telephone & Electronics
HR	Heart Rate
IAN	Incident Area Network
IC	Incident Commander

ICT	Information and Communication Technology
IEEE	Institute of Electrical and Electronics Engineers
INMARSAT	International Maritime Satellite
ISDN	Integrated Services Digital Network
LAN	Local Area Network
LED	Light Emitting Diode
LEO	Low Earth Orbit
LOS	Line of Sight
MANET	Management of Catastrophic Events by using Autonomous Sensor Networks
MCI	Mass Casualty Incident
MIO	Medical Incident Officer
NASA	National Aeronautics and Space Administration
NFC	Near Field Communication
NLOS	Non Line of Sight
NMEA	National Marine Electronics Association
PCB	Printed Board Circuit
PDA	Personal Digital Assitant
PED	Prehospital Emergency Doctors
PI	Perfusion Index
PIL	Processor in the Loop
RFID	Radio Frequency Identification
RSSI	Received Signal Strenght Indication
SECOSERV	Secure Communication and Information Platform for Mass Casualty Incident Scenarios
SOGRO	Instant Recovery in Major Accident
SpO2	Pulse Oximetry
START	Simple Triage And Rapid Treatment
TETRA	Terrestrial Trunked Radio
TI	Texas Instruments
UN	United Nations
WAN	Wide Area Network
WIISARD	Wireless Internet Information System for Medical Response
WISECOM	Wireless Infrastructure over Satellite for Emergency Communications
WLAN	Wireless Local Area Network
WPAN	Wireless Personal Area Networks

Literature and References

[AEMK12] C. Adler, L. Erfurt, A. Metz and M. Krüsmann. "Schlussbericht e-Triage: Elektronische Betroffenenerfassung in Katastrophenfällen". Ludwig-Maximilians-Universität–München. November 2012

[AF12] P. Aitken and G. FitzGerald. "Disaster triage: Evidence, consistency and standard practice". Emergency Medicine Australasia, vol. 24(3): pp. 222–224. 2012

[AI08] S. Ahson and M. Ilyas. RFID Handbook: Applications, Technology, Security, and Privacy, Taylor & Francis2008

[AKGM+11] C. Adler, M. Krüsmann, T. Greiner-Mai, A. Donner et al. "IT-Supported Management of Mass Casualty Incidents : The e-Triage Project". Proceedings of the 8th International ISCRAM Conference–Lisbon, p. Vol. 1. May 2011

[BCC+11] M. Berioli, J. M. Chaves, N. Courville, P. Boutry et al. "WISECOM: A rapidly deployable satellite backhauling system for emergency situations". International Journal of Satellite Communications and Networking, vol. 29(5): pp. 419–440. 2011

[BCK+07] C. Buono, T. Chan, J. Killeen, R. Huang et al. "Comparison of the effectiveness of wireless electronic tracking devices versus traditional paper systems to track victims in a large scale disaster". AMIA Annu Symp Proc. 2007, vol. 886

[BCW07a] M. Berioli, N. Courville and M. Werner. "Emergency communications over satellite: the WISECOM approach". Mobile and Wireless Communications Summit, 2007. 16th IST, IEEE2007, pp. 1–5

[BCW07b] M. Berioli, N. Courville and M. Werner. "Integrating satellite and terrestrial technologies for emergency communications: the WISECOM project". QShine 2007 Workshop: Satellite/Terrestrial Interworking, ACM2007, p. 2

[BGD+06] S. W. Brown, M. S. W. G. Griswold, B. Demchak, B. A. L. A. Lenert et al. "Middleware for Reliable Mobile Medical Workflow Support in Disaster Settings". Symposium A Quarterly Journal In Modern Foreign Literatures–San Diego, California, pp. 309–313. 2006

[BKH+09] H. Bail, C. Kleber, N. Haas, P. Fischer et al. "Verteilungsplanung von Verletzten beim MANV oder Katastrophenfall". Der Unfallchirurg, vol. 112(10): pp. 870–877. 2009

[BKS96] M. Benson, K. L. Koenig and C. H. Schultz. "Disaster triage: START, then SAVE a new method of dynamic triage for victims of a catastrophic earthquake". Prehospital and disaster medicine, vol. 11(02): pp. 117–124. 1996

[Bla04] C. R. Blagg. "Triage: Napoleon to the present day". Journal of nephrology, vol. 17: pp. 629–632. 2004

[BU12] A. Bolz and W. Urbaszek. Technik in der Kardiologie: Eine interdisziplinäre Darstellung für Ingenieure und Mediziner, Springer Verlag2012

[CARQ01] M. F. Cabrera, M. T. Arredondo, A. Rodriguez and J. Quiroga. "Mobile technologies in the management of disasters: the results of a telemedicine solution." Proceedings of the AMIA Symposium, American Medical Informatics Association2001, p. 86

[CBP+09] D. W. Curtis, J. Bailey, E. J. Pino, T. Stair et al. "Using ambient intelligence for physiological monitoring". Journal of Ambient Intelligence and Smart Environments, vol. 1(2): pp. 129–142. 2009

[CdAG13] A. Castanheira de Almeida Guerra. Design and development of a new TRIAGE concept for the rapid classification and localization of victims during MCI. Master's thesis, Karlsruher Institute für Technologie. 2013

[CES82] R. Cowley, S. Edelstein and Silverstein. Mass Casualties, a Lessons Learned Approach: Accidents, Civil Disorders, Natural Disasters, Terrorism, U.S. Department of

Transportation, National Highway Traffic Safety Administration1982

[CFY02] M. D. Christian, J. C. Farmer and B. P. Young. "Disaster triage and allocation of scarce resources". Fundamentals of Disaster ManagementSociety of Critical Care Medicine–Mount Prospect–IL. 2002

[CGP+12] O. Chipara, W. G. Griswold, A. N. Plymoth, R. Huang et al. "WIISARD: a measurement study of network properties and protocol reliability during an emergency response". Proceedings of the 10th international conference on Mobile systems, applications, and services, ACM2012, pp. 407–420

[CK10] J. Campbell and F. Kühl. Präklinische Traumatologie, Pearson Studium2010. URL http://books.google.de/books?id=AhypfiOwapUC

[CKGL04] T. C. Chan, J. Killeen, W. Griswold and L. Lenert. "Information technology and emergency medical care during disasters". Academic emergency medicine, vol. 11(11): pp. 1229–1236. 2004

[CM05] D. C. Cone and D. S. MacMillan. "Mass-casualty Triage Systems: A Hint of Science". Academic Emergency Medicine, vol. 12(8): pp. 739–741. 2005

[CM06] R. Carella and S. McGrath. "ARTEMIS personal area networks for emergency remote triage and information management". Proceedings of the 3rd. international ISCRAM conference, pp. 592–597. 2006

[CMV12] T. Case, C. Morrison and A. Vuylsteke. "The clinical application of mobile technology to disaster medicine". Prehospital and disaster medicine, vol. 27(05): pp. 473–480. 2012

[Cow82] R. A. Cowley. "Mass casualty needs–Baltimore, Maryland Mass Casualties: A Lessons Learned Approach." Proceedings of the First International Assembly on Emergency Medical Services, pp. 141–145. June 1982

[CS09] A.-K. Chandra-Sekaran. A location aware wireless sensor network for assisting emergency response to disasters. Ph.D. thesis. Karlsruher Institut für Technologie (KIT), Diss.

[CSFK+08] A.-K. Chandra-Sekaran, G. Flaig, C. Kunze, W. Stork et al. "Efficient resource estimation during mass casualty emergency response based on a location aware disaster aid network". Wireless Sensor Networks, Springer2008, pp. 205–220

[CSK10] A.-K. Chandra-Sekaran and C. Kunze. "Self-Organizing ZigBee Network and Bayesian Filter Based Patient Localization Approaches for Disaster Management". International Journal On Advances in Intelligent Systems, vol. 2(4): pp. 446–456. 2010

[CTD+02] J. R. Clarke, S. Z. Trooskin, P. J. Doshi, L. Greenwald et al. "Time to laparotomy for intra-abdominal bleeding from trauma does affect survival for delays up to 90 minutes". Journal of Trauma and Acute Care Surgery, vol. 52(3): pp. 420–425. 2002

[CU05] V. Chan and S. Underwood. "A single-chip pulsoximeter design using the MSP430". Tech. rep. Texas Instruments 2005

[DAGM12] A. Donner, R. Arlt and T. Greiner-Mai. "Jenseits von Papier und Sprache. Anmerkungen zur MANV-Bewältigung mit digitaler Informations-und Kommunikationstechnik". 1. Symposium ICT in der Notfallmedizin (NotIT). German Medical Science, Rauischholzhausen. 2012, pp. 73–79

[DEA+11] A. Donner, S. Erl, C. Adler, A. Metz et al. "Projekt e-Triage: Datenmanagement für die elektronische Betroffenenerfassung und Akzeptanz bei Rettungskräften". Beiträge der 41. Jahrestagung der Gesellschaft fÃijr Informatik e.V. (GI)–Berlin. 2011

[Del09] W. J. Delaney. "Mobile temporary incident area network for local communications interoperability". Mar. 2009

[DGL07] B. Demchak, W. G. Griswold and L. A. Lenert. "Data quality for situational awareness during mass-casualty events". AMIA annual symposium proceedings, American Medical Informatics Association2007, vol. 2007, p. 176

[EFK13] N. Ellebrecht, K. Feldmeier and S. Kaufmann. "IT's about more than speed. The impact of IT on the management of mass casualty incidents in Germany". Proceedings of the 10th international ISCRAM conference. Baden-Baden. 2013, pp. 1–10

[EL12] N. Ellebrecht and L. Latasch. "Vorsichtung durch Rettungsassistenten auf der Großübung SOGRO MANV 500". Notfall+ Rettungsmedizin, vol. 15(1): pp. 58–64. 2012

[ER02] A. El-Rabbany. Introduction to GPS: The Global Positioning System. Artech House mobile communications series, Artech House2002

[FL] E. A. Fry and L. A. Lenert. "MASCAL: RFID tracking of patients, staff and equipment to enhance hospital response to mass casualty events". AMIA Annual Symposium Proceedings. American Medical Informatics Association, vol. 2005, p. 261

[FMB07] K. A. Farmer, S. P. McGrath and G. T. Blike. "An experimental architecture for observation of triage related decision making". Engineering in Medicine and Biology Society, EMBS–29th Annual International Conference, IEEE2007, pp. 1774–1777

[FWC+08] E. H. Fazli, M. Werner, N. Courville, M. Berioli et al. "Integrated GSM/WiFi backhauling over satellite: Flexible solution for emergency communications". Vehicular Technology Conference, IEEE2008, pp. 2962–2966

[Gar03] A. Garner. "Documentation and tagging of casualties in multiple casualty incidents". Emergency Medicine, vol. 15(5-6): pp. 475–479. 2003

[GAR+05] B. Gorgaß, F. Ahnefeld, R. Rossi, H. Lippert et al. Rettungsassistent und Rettungssanitäter, Springer2005

[GAR+07] B. Gorgaß, F. Ahnefeld, R. Rossi, H. Lippert et al. Das Rettungsdienst-Lehrbuch, Springer Berlin–Heidelberg2007

[GB99] V. Garshnek and F. M. Burkle. "Applications of telemedicine and telecommunications to disaster medicine historical and future perspectives". Journal of the American Medical Informatics Association, vol. 6(1): pp. 26–37. 1999

[GGW+06] T. Gao, D. Greenspan, M. Welsh, R. Juang et al. "Vital signs monitoring and patient tracking over a wireless network". Engineering in Medicine and Biology Society EMBS 2005 27th Annual International Conference, IEEE2006, pp. 102–105

[GLHS01] A. Garner, A. Lee, K. Harrison and C. H. Schultz. "Comparative analysis of multiple-casualty incident triage algorithms". Annals of emergency medicine, vol. 38(5): pp. 541–548. 2001

[GMD10] T. Greiner-Mai and A. Donner. "Data Management in Mass Casualty Incidents: The e-Triage Project." GI Jahrestagung (2). 2010, pp. 192–198

[GMS+07a] T. Gao, T. Massey, M. Sarrafzadeh, L. Selavo et al. "Participatory user centered design techniques for a large scale ad-hoc health information system". Proceedings of the 1st ACM SIGMOBILE international workshop on Systems and networking support for healthcare and assisted living environments, ACM2007, pp. 43–48

[GMS+07b] T. Gao, T. Massey, L. Selavo, D. Crawford et al. "The advanced health and disaster aid network: A light-weight wireless medical system for triage". Biomedical Circuits and Systems, IEEE Transactions on, vol. 1(3): pp. 203–216. 2007

[Gon13] M. Goniewicz. "Effect of Military Conflicts on the Formation of Emergency Medical Services Systems Worldwide". Academic Emergency Medicine, vol. 20(5): pp. 507–513. 2013

[GSMF05] M. Gaynor, M. Seltzer, S. Moulton and J. Freedman. "A dynamic, data-driven, decision support system for emergency medical services". International Conference on Computational ScienceâĂŞ-ICCS, Springer2005, pp. 703–711

[HCP08] D. B. Hoyt, R. Coimbra and B. M. Potenza. "Trauma systems, triage, and transport". Trauma, 6th edition. New York, NY, McGraw-Hill, pp. 57–82. 2008

[HHMS98] T. J. Hodgetts, J. Hall, I. Maconochie and C. Smart. "Pediatric triage tape". Pre-Hospital Immediate Care, vol. 2: pp. 155–9. 1998

[HRR+14] S. Heuer, D. Rodriguez, S. Ruß, B. Weber et al. "Ein sensorgestÃijtztes Kommunikations- und Informationssystem zur UnterstÃijtzung von Versorgung und Organisation in MANV-Szenarien". e-Health, Informations- und Kommunikationstechnologien im Gesundheitswesen, pp. 82–94. 2014

[HUY11] T. Higashino, A. Uchiyama and K. Yasumoto. "eTriage: A wireless communication service platform for advanced rescue operations". Proc. of ACM Workshop on Internet of Things and Service Patforms (IoTSP). 2011

[Ina11a] V. S. Inampudi. A real time web based electronic triage, resource allocation and hospital dispatch system for emergency. Ph.D. thesis, University of Massachusetts Amherst. 2011

[Ina11b] V. S. Inampudi. A real time web based electronic triage, resource allocation and hospital dispatch system for emergency. Ph.D. thesis, University of Massachusetts Amherst. 2011

[ISOF06] S. Inoue, A. Sonoda, K. I. Oka and S. Fujisaki. "Triage with RFID tags". Pervasive Health Conference and Workshops, 2006, IEEE2006, pp. 1–7

[JGK+08] L. C. JatobÃą, U. Grossmann, C. Kunze, J. Ottenbacher et al. "Context-aware mobile health monitoring: Evaluation of different pattern recognition methods for classification of physical activity". Engineering in Medicine and Biology Society, 2008. EMBS 2008. 30th Annual International Conference of the IEEE, IEEE2008, pp. 5250–5253

[JGO+08] L. C. Jatobá, U. Großmann, J. Ottenbacher, S. Härtel et al. "Obtaining energy expenditure and physical activity from acceleration signals for context-aware evaluation of cardiovascular parameters". IV Latin American Congress on Biomedical Engineering 2007, Bioengineering Solutions for Latin America Health, Springer2008, pp. 475–479

[JRG+12] J. Jokela, M. R, D. Gryth, H. Nilsson et al. "Increased situation awareness in major incidentsâĂŤradio frequency identification (RFID) technique: A promising tool". Prehospital and disaster medicine, vol. 27(01): pp. 81–87. 2012

[KAGL96] K. Kennedy, R. V. Aghababian, L. Gans and C. P. Lewis. "Triage: techniques and applications in decisionmaking". Annals of Emergency Medicine, vol. 28(2): pp. 136–144. 1996

[KCB+06] J. P. Killeen, T. C. Chan, C. Buono, W. G. Griswold et al. "A wireless first responder handheld device for rapid triage, patient assessment and documentation during mass casualty incidents". AMIA annual symposium proceedings, American Medical Informatics Association2006, vol. 2006, p. 429

[KN07] K. R. Klein and N. E. Nagel. "Mass medical evacuation: Hurricane Katrina and nursing experiences at the New Orleans airport". Disaster Management & Response, vol. 5(2): pp. 56–61. 2007

[KNO11] H. Kojima, K. Nagahashi and K.-i. Okada. "Proposal of the Disaster-Relief Training System Using the Electronic Triage Tag". International Conference on Advanced Information Networking and Applications (AINA), IEEE2011, pp. 256–263

[KRS+09] C. Kunze, D. Rodriguez, L. Shammas, A.-K. Chandra-Sekaran et al. "Nutzung von Sensornetzwerken und mobilen Informationsgeräten für die Situationserfassung und die Prozessunterstützung bei Massenanfällen von Verletzten." GI Jahrestagung. 2009, pp. 1465–1478

[Kun] C. Kunze. Ubiquitous healthcare: Anwendung ubiquitärer Informationstechnologien im Telemonitoring. Ph.D. thesis, Karlsruhe, Univ., Diss., 2005

[KWF12] B. Käser, B. Weber and S. Frederik. "Die Patientenanhängetasche/-karte in der medizinischen Gefahrenabwehr The triage card used in the medical hazard prevention". NotIT 2012, 1. Symposium ICT in der Notfallmedizin, pp. 63–66. June 2012

[LB05] A. Lima and J. Bakker. "Noninvasive monitoring of peripheral perfusion". Intensive care medicine, vol. 31(10): pp. 1316–1326. 2005

[LCG+06] L. Lenert, T. C. Chan, W. Griswold, J. Killeen et al. "Wireless internet information system for medical response in disasters (wiisard)". AMIA annual symposium proceedings, American Medical Informatics Association2006, vol. 2006, p. 1192

[LDWS12] R. Lawatschek, S. Düsterwald, C. Wirth and T. Schröder. "Alarm: A Modular IT Solution to Support and Evaluate Mass Casualty Incident (MCI) Management". Proceedings of the 9th International ISCRAM Conference. 2012

[Lee10] C. H. Lee. "Disaster and Mass Casualty Triage". Virtual Mentor–American Medical Association, vol. 12(6): p. 466. 2010

[LH14] D. Larrey and R. Hall. Memoirs of Military Surgery, and Campaigns of the French Armies, on the Rhine, in Corsica, Catalonia, Egypt, and Syria; at Boulogne, Ulm, and Austerlitz; in Saxony, Prussia, Poland, Spain, and Austria, vol. 1 of Memoirs of Military Surgery, Ed. Joseph Cushing1814

[LKG+11] L. A. Lenert, D. Kirsh, W. G. Griswold, C. Buono et al. "Design and evaluation of a wireless electronic health records system for field care in mass casualty settings". Journal of the American Medical Informatics Association, vol. 18(6): pp. 842–852. 2011

[LM32] D. LARREY and J. MERCER. Surgical Memoirs of the Campaigns of Russia, Germany, and France, vol. 4, Carey & Lea1832

[LMFj+04] K. Lorincz, D. J. Malan, T. Fulford-jones, A. Clavel et al. "Sensor Networks for Emergency Response: Challenges and Opportunities". Pervasive Computing IEEE, pp. 16–23. 2004

[LSC+08] E. B. Lerner, R. B. Schwartz, P. L. Coule, E. S. Weinstein et al. "Mass casualty triage: an evaluation of the data and development of a proposed national guideline". Disaster medicine and public health preparedness, vol. 2(1): pp. 25–34. 2008

[MB07] B. S. Manoj and A. H. Baker. "Communication challenges in emergency response". Communications of the ACM, vol. 50(3): pp. 51–53. 2007

[MCMYC11] A. Martín-Campillo, R. Martí, E. Yoneki and J. Crowcroft. "Electronic triage tag and opportunistic networks in disasters". Proceedings of the Special Workshop on Internet and Disasters, ACM2011, p. 6

[MFJWM04] D. Malan, T. Fulford-Jones, M. Welsh and S. Moulton. "Codeblue: An ad hoc sensor network infrastructure for emergency medical care". International workshop on wearable and implantable body sensor networks. 2004, vol. 5

[MGB+06] T. Massey, T. Gao, D. Bernstein, A. Husain et al. "Pervasive triage: Towards ubiquitous, real-time monitoring of vital signs for pre-hospital applications". Proceedings of the International Workshop on Ubiquitous Computing for Pervasive Healthcare. 2006

[MGW+03] S. McGrath, E. Grigg, S. Wendelken, G. Blike et al. "Artemis: A vision for remote triage and emergency management information integration". Dartmouth University, p. 9. 2003

[MGW+06] T. Massey, T. Gao, M. Welsh, J. H. Sharp et al. "The design of a decentralized electronic triage system". AMIA annual symposium proceedings, American Medical Informatics Association2006, pp. 544–548

[MIS+12] T. Mizumoto, S. Imazu, W. Sun, N. Shibata et al. "Emergency medical support system for visualizing locations and vital signs of patients in Mass Casualty Incident". Pervasive Computing and Communications Workshops (PERCOM Workshops), 2012 IEEE International Conference on, IEEE2012, pp. 740–745

[Mit08] G. W. Mitchell. "A brief history of triage". Disaster medicine and public health preparedness, vol. 2(1): pp. 4–7. 2008

[MJT00] M. Morin, J. Jenvald and M. Thorstensson. "Computer-supported visualization of rescue operations". Safety Science, vol. 35(1): pp. 3–27. 2000

[MSYI11] T. Mizumoto, W. Sun, K. Yasumoto and M. Ito. "Transportation scheduling method for patients in mci using electronic triage tag". eTELEMED 2011, The Third International Conference on eHealth, Telemedicine and Social Medicine. 2011, pp. 156–163

[MW12] S. A. Mathias Wilhelm, Eva Burneleit. "Tactical Information Visualization for Operation Managers in Mass Casualty Incidents". Proceedings of the Workshop on AmI for Crisis Management (AmI4CM 2012), CEUR-WS.org2012, vol. 953 of CEUR Workshop Proceedings

[NAC+11] S. Nestler, E. Artinger, T. Coskun, T. Endres et al. "RFID based patient registration in mass casualty incidents". GMS Medizinische Informatik, Biometrie und Epidemiologie, vol. 7: pp. 1–9. 2011

[NG99a] A. Nocera and A. Garner. "Australian disaster triage: a colour maze in the Tower of Babel." The Australian and New Zealand journal of surgery, vol. 69(8): pp. 598–602. Aug. 1999

[NG99b] A. Nocera and A. Garner. "An Australian mass casualty incident triage system for the future based upon triage mistakes of the past: the Homebush Triage Standard". Australian and New Zealand journal of surgery, vol. 69(8): pp. 603–608. 1999

[NK07] S. Nestler and G. Klinker. "Using mobile hand-held computers in disasters". UbiComp Workshop on Interaction with Ubiquitous Wellness and Healthcare Applications (UbiWell). 2007

[oHS08] U. D. of Homeland Security. "National Incident Management System". URL http://www.dhs.comhttp://www.fema.gov/media-library/assets/documents/25422. 2008

[PD10] R. Powers and E. Daily. International Disaster Nursing, Cambridge University Press2010

[Pea05] R. Pearce. "Historical developments in casualty evacuation and triage". Australian Military Medicine, vol. 14(2): p. 54.

[PRAD08] S. A. Paul, M. Reddy, J. Abraham and C. DeFlitch. "The usefulness of information and communication technologies in crisis response". AMIA Annual Symposium Proceedings, American Medical Informatics Association2008, p. 561

[PRS07] O. Peters, K. Runggaldier and T. Schlechtriemen. "Algorithmen im Rettungsdienst". Notfall+ Rettungsmedizin, vol. 10(3): pp. 229–236. 2007

[RAV+10] M. Rehn, J. E. Andersen, T. Vigerust, A. J. Krüger et al. "A concept for major incident triage: full-scaled simulation feasibility study". BMC emergency medicine, vol. 10(1): p. 17. 2010

[RHG+14] D. Rodriguez, S. Heuer, A. Guerra, W. Stork et al. "Towards automatic sensor-based triage for individual remote monitoring during mass casualty incidents". 2014 IEEE International Conference on Bioinformatics and Biomedicine–Belfast, UK, IEEE2014, pp. 544–551

[RHKW11] D. Rodriguez, S. Heuer, C. Kunze and B. Weber. "Management of mass casualty of incidents using an autonomous sensor network". 14th International Symposium on Wireless Personal Multimedia Communications (WPMC)–Brest, France, IEEE2011, pp. 1–5

[Rom11] D. L. Romig. "The JumpSTART Pediatric MCI Triage Tool and other pediatric disaster and emergency medicine resources". URL http://www.jumpstarttriage.com. 2011

[RPA+09] M. C. Reddy, S. A. Paul, J. Abraham, M. McNeese et al. "Challenges to effective crisis management: using information and communication technologies to coordinate emergency medical services and emergency department teams". International journal of medical informatics, vol. 78(4): pp. 259–269. 2009

[RR92] C. J. Runcie and W. Reeve. "Is portable capnometry useful during transport of the critically ill?" Journal of Clinical Monitoring and Computing, vol. 8(3): pp. 250–250. 1992

[RYS+12] D. S. Radvinsky, R. S. Yoon, P. J. Schmitt, C. J. Prestigiacomo et al. "Evolution and development of the Advanced Trauma Life Support (ATLS) protocol: a historical perspective". Orthopedics, vol. 35(4): pp. 305–11. 2012

[SCL+05] V. Shnayder, B.-r. Chen, K. Lorincz, T. R. F. Jones et al. "Sensor networks for medical care". SenSys. 2005, vol. 5, pp. 314–314

[SGB+06] J. D. Schenker, S. Goldstein, J. Braun, A. Werner et al. "Triage accuracy at a multiple casualty incident disaster drill: the Emergency Medical Service, Fire Department of New York City experience". Journal of burn care & research, vol. 27(5): pp. 570–575. 2006

[SHS+11] K. Sakanushi, T. Hieda, T. Shiraishi, Y. Ode et al. "Electronic Triage System: Casualties Monitoring System in the Disaster Scene". P2P, Parallel, Grid, Cloud and Internet Computing (3PGCIC), 2011 International Conference on, IEEE2011, pp. 317–322

[SHS+13] K. Sakanushi, T. Hieda, T. Shiraishi, Y. Ode et al. "Electronic triage system for continuously monitoring casualties at disaster scenes". Journal of Ambient Intelligence and Humanized Computing, vol. 4(5): pp. 547–558. 2013

[Sid12] E. Siddiqui. "Emergency Triage: Extend of our knowledge". JPMA–Emergency. 2012

[SLZ+06] P. N. Skandalakis, P. Lainas, O. Zoras, J. E. Skandalakis et al. "To afford the wounded speedy assistance: Dominique Jean Larrey and Napoleon". World journal of surgery, vol. 30(8): pp. 1392–1399. 2006

[Sob13] R. Sobar. Entwicklung und Evaluation eines neuen eingebetteten Systems zur Triage von Patienten während MANV Szenarien. Master's thesis, Karlsruher Institute für Technologie. 2013

[spa] "Advanced hybrid satellite and terrestrial system architecture for emergency mobile communications". 26th International Communications Satellite Systems Condference, AIAA–San Diego

[U.N92] U.N. "An Overview of Disaster Management". Tech. Rep. 2nd., United Nations, Sweden. 1992

[Vem04] T. Vemmer. The Management of Mass Casualty Incidends in Germany, Books on Demand2004

[VTEC86] J. S. Vayer, R. Ten Eyck and M. Cowan. "New concepts in triage". Annals of emergency medicine, vol. 15(8): pp. 927–930. 1986

[WDH+10] S. Waddington, D. Dodman, J. Hardoy, Johnson, D. Sattertwaite et al. "World Disasters Report 2010". Tech. rep., International Federation of the Red Cross and Red Crescent Societies, Geneva, Switzerland. URL www.ifrc.org. 2010

[Web09] J. Webster. Medical Instrumentation Application and Design, 4th Edition, Wiley Global Education2009

[WLA12] "IEEE 802.11: WIRELESS PERSONAL AREA NETWORKS (PANs)". URL http://standards.ieee.org/about/get/802/802.11.html. 2012

[WMB03] S. M. Wendelken, S. P. McGrath and G. T. Blike. "A medical assessment algorithm for automated remote triage". Proceedings of the 25th Annual International Conference of the IEEE Engineering in Medicine and Biology Society, IEEE2003, vol. 4, pp. 3630–3633

[WMBA04] S. Wendelken, S. McGrath, G. Blike and M. Akay. "The feasibility of using a forehead reflectance pulse oximeter for automated remote triage". Proceedings of the IEEE 30th Annual Bioengineering Conference, IEEE2004, pp. 180–181

[WPA05] "IEEE 802.15.1 WIRELESS PERSONAL AREA NETWORKS (PANs)". URL http://standards.ieee.org/about/get/802/802.15.html. 2005

[ZIG14] "Zigbee Alliance". URL http://www.zigbee.org. 2014

Publications

[HMFO09] S. Heuer, D. R. Martinez, S. Fuhrhop and J. Ottenbacher. "Motion artefact correction for capacitive ECG measurement". Biomedical Circuits and Systems Conference, 2009. BioCAS 2009. IEEE, IEEE2009, pp. 113–116

[HRR+14] S. Heuer, D. Rodriguez, S. Ruß, B. Weber et al. "Ein sensorgestütztes Kommunikations- und Informationssystem zur Unterstützung von Versorgung und Organisation in MANV-Szenarien". e-Health, Informations- und Kommunikationstechnologien im Gesundheitswesen, pp. 82–94. 2014

[KRS+09] C. Kunze, D. Rodriguez, L. Shammas, A.-K. Chandra-Sekaran et al. "Nutzung von Sensornetzwerken und mobilen Informationsgeräten für die Situationserfassung und die Prozessunterstützung bei Massenanfällen von Verletzten." GI Jahrestagung. 2009, pp. 1465–1478

[RHG+14] D. Rodriguez, S. Heuer, A. Guerra, W. Stork et al. "Towards automatic sensor-based triage for individual remote monitoring during mass casualty incidents". 2014 IEEE International Conference on Bioinformatics and Biomedicine–Belfast, UK, IEEE2014, pp. 544–551

[RHKW11] D. Rodriguez, S. Heuer, C. Kunze and B. Weber. "Management of mass casualty of incidents using an autonomous sensor network". 14th International Symposium on Wireless Personal Multimedia Communications (WPMC)–Brest, France, IEEE2011, pp. 1–5

[Rod14] D. Rodriguez. "A novel platform for automatic triage and rapid localization of patients during mass casualty incidents". 11th International ISCRAM Conference–University Park, Pennsylvania, USA, IEEE2014

[RWG$^+$] S. Ruß, B. Weber, S. Graffy, D. Rodriguez et al. "Kritisch oder unkritisch? Automatische Vorsichtung beim MANV". Rettungsdienst, vol. 36(12): p. 26

Supervised Students Theses

[Ale12] I. Alesanco. TrinkTracker–Platform for the daily and individual monitoring of water and liquid consumption in residences for the elderly. Master's thesis, Karlsruher Institute für Technologie. 2012

[CdAG13] A. Castanheira de Almeida Guerra. Design and development of a new TRIAGE concept for the rapid classification and localization of victims during MCI. Master's thesis, Karlsruher Institute für Technologie. 2013

[Gal14] M. Gall. Konzeption und Evaluation einer mobilen Sensorplattform zur Überwachung der körperlichen und emotionalen Belastung von Rettungskräften bei Massenunfällen, Bachelor's thesis, Karlsruher Institute für Technologie. 2014

[InR14] A. Ibañez Rodríguez. Conception and evaluation of a new TRIAGE algorithm based on the processing of vital and physiological parameters. Master's thesis, Karlsruher Institute für Technologie. 2014

[Kur14] M. Kurth. Konzeption und Evaluationeines Algorithmus zur Bewertung und Klassifizierung der physiologischen Belastung von Rettungskräften bei Massenunfällen. Master's thesis, Karlsruher Institute für Technologie. 2014

[SFFD11] M. Schmelze, E. Fiedler, S. Feuer and R. D. TrinkTracker, Ambient Assisted Living (AAL), Seminar Wissensmanagement, Karlsruher Institute für Technologie. 2011

[Sha10] K. Shakeryan. Development of a Mobile Pulse Transient Time Measuring System. Master's thesis, Universität Karlsruhe (TH). 2010

[Sob13] R. Sobar. Entwicklung und Evaluation eines neuen eingebetteten Systems zur Triage von Patienten während MANV Szenarien. Master's thesis, Karlsruher Institute für Technologie. 2013

[SWO11] K. Schultze-Westrum and I. Omurok. Dekubitus Assitenz, Ambient Assisted Living (AAL), Seminar Wissensmanagement, Karlsruher Institute für Technologie. 2011

Resume

Personal Information	
Name	José David Rodríguez Martínez
Birthday	24.05.1982
Birthplace	Mexico City
Nationality	mexican
Education	
10/2005 - 11/2008	M. Sc. in Electrical Engineering specialized in Information and Communication Technologies University of Karlsruhe (TH), Germany
08/2000 - 05/2005	B. Sc. in Mechatronics specialized in Control Engineering and Automation Monterrey Institute of Technology and Higher Education, Mexico
08/1997 - 05/2000	High school at Monterrey Institute of Technology and Higher Education, Mexico
Work Experience	
from 11/2014	System Engineer in the Area of Ultrasonic Sensors for Comfort and Driving Assitance Systems Valeo Schalter und Sensoren GmbH, Bietigheim-Bissigen, Germany
12/2008 - 09/2014	Research Scientist in the Department of Embedded Systems and Sensors Engineering Forschungszentrum Informatik am Karlsruher Institut für Technologie, Karlsruhe, Germany
10/2007 - 03/2008	Industrial Internship in the Area of Building Technologies Siemens AG, Karlsruhe, Germany
03/2007 - 08/2007	Industrial Internship in the Area of Automotive Radars Siemens VDO Automotive AG, Lindau, Germany